The Global War on Tobacco

The Global War on Tobacco

Mapping the World's First Public Health Treaty

HEATHER WIPFLI

Johns Hopkins University Press

Baltimore

© 2015 Johns Hopkins University Press
All rights reserved. Published 2015
Printed in the United States of America on acid-free paper
2   4   6   8   9   7   5   3   1

Johns Hopkins University Press
2715 North Charles Street
Baltimore, Maryland 21218-4363
www.press.jhu.edu

Library of Congress Cataloging-in-Publication Data
Wipfli, Heather, 1976–, author.
The global war on tobacco : mapping the world's first public health treaty /
Heather Wipfli.
p. ; cm.
Includes bibliographical references and index.
ISBN 978-1-4214-1683-0 (pbk. : alk. paper) — ISBN 1-4214-1683-2 (pbk. : alk.
paper) — ISBN 978-1-4214-1684-7 (electronic) — ISBN 1-4214-1684-0 (electronic)
I. Title.
[DNLM: 1. WHO Framework Convention on Tobacco Control (2003) 2. Smoking—
legislation & jurisprudence. 3. International Cooperation. 4. Smoking—prevention
& control. 5. Tobacco Industry—legislation & jurisprudence. 6. Tobacco Use
Disorder—prevention & control. WM 33.1]
HD9130.5
338.4'76797—dc23   2014036893

A catalog record for this book is available from the British Library.

*Special discounts are available for bulk purchases of this book. For more information,
please contact Special Sales at 410-516-6936 or specialsales@press.jhu.edu.*

Johns Hopkins University Press uses environmentally friendly book materials,
including recycled text paper that is composed of at least 30 percent post-consumer
waste, whenever possible.

CONTENTS

Few of my childhood memories are as potent as those of sitting on my paternal grandfather's lap as he sat hunch-backed, gasping for air through his oxygen machine. Never one to offer an easy smile, my paternal grandfather was a grumpy, elderly man facing his own physical demise—a demise caused by his lifelong addiction to cigarettes. My grandfather was angry. He was angry that his golden years were stolen from him after he had worked hard his entire life, fighting first for his country and then for his family. He was a fervent supporter of tobacco control efforts and detested the tobacco industry with all his heart. His anger and illness transferred these same feelings to his entire family, myself included.

Ironically, another strong memory I have from childhood was when my grandmother bought a small wooden sign to hang in her kitchen that read No Smoking. It was pretty, blue and white, and very unassuming. She mused for days over whether to hang it and whether it was appropriate to ask her guests not to smoke in her house—even when the presence of smoke could possibly cause her husband respiratory failure. Thirty years later such social concerns seem crazy in the United States. Smoking norms have dramatically changed thanks to the hard work of countless tobacco control leaders in the United States and around the world.

Although I had personal experience with tobacco-caused disease and death (so many of us do), I never anticipated that I would dedicate my career to tobacco control. I set off to study international politics and moved to Geneva, Switzerland, after graduation from college with every intention of practicing global politics. Working within diverse cultures and experiencing our common humanity has always excited me. In my mind, however, international politics was largely limited to war and peace. Just by circumstance, I landed my first internship at the World Health Organization on the Policy Action Coordination team then headed by a rising star named Derek Yach. Derek would later offer me (a starving student) an administrative job with the Tobacco Free Initiative (TFI) assisting with preparations for the first Framework Convention on Tobacco Control (FCTC) working group. The atmosphere in TFI at the time was electrifying. There was a sense that we were breaking the rules of the game and anything was possible. The general approach was to "ask for forgiveness rather than permission." I jumped into the work headfirst and quickly became a technical officer on the FCTC team under the leadership of Douglas Bettcher. I remained at TFI for three years while the treaty was negotiated.

That experience gave me an insider's perspective on the FCTC process. I'll never forget the long nights at Geneva's International Conference Center, sitting dumbfounded with a handful of the world's greatest lawyers and trying helplessly to decode the mess of overlapping proposals that the chair's draft had become. I will also never forget the passion and brilliance of so many that made the FCTC a reality.

Tobacco control has a way of sucking people into the work. I left TFI before the negotiations came to a conclusion and moved to the Institute for Global Tobacco Control at the Johns Hopkins Bloomberg School of Public Health, where I served as project director for the next eight years. In this position I was able to observe the FCTC process from afar and take a more academic approach toward its evaluation, including finishing my PhD on the role of diffusion, norms, and governance in global tobacco control.

This book is a culmination of these experiences. I have attempted to remain scholarly and objective in my analysis of the process, although it is safe to say that I am a firm believer in the FCTC process, if for no other reason than its fundamental acknowledgment that global health is political and, at times, requires a political response. In other words, there is a place for people like me in global health. Shortly after I joined TFI full time, and just after I completed my master's degree in international politics at the Graduate Institute of International and Development Studies at the University of Geneva, I was invited out to lunch by a fellow recent alum. He had been hired by an international consulting firm and was working on a contract with a consortium of alcohol companies. They were, in my colleague's words, petrified by the progress of the FCTC and believed that they would be the next target. He admitted to me that he was responsible for collecting intelligence on the process to help them prepare a defense. Sitting here in my office 15 years later, it is shocking to me that alcohol companies have largely been successful in their tactics to avoid similar accountability and forestall global regulation. I hope that this book will help others in global health understand the FCTC process and motivate them to further investigate how international legal instruments can be used for other areas of global health, especially those plagued by unfettered corporate activity and greed.

Of course, a book such as this is not developed in isolation. Evidence and insight for this book came from all corners of the globe and involved countless people from all walks of life. I wish to first thank Jonathan Samet, my primary research collaborator and mentor for nearly 15 years. He has provided me a professional environment that has allowed me to learn and grow, and he has never turned down an opportunity to read and edit my writing. Past and present members of TFI provided feedback on early chapter drafts, and Laurent Huber, director of the Framework Convention Alliance, provided both input and access to images. Menchi Velasco with the Southeast Asian Tobacco Control Alliance helped set up my interviews in Thailand and ensured that I never got out of Thailand without singing karaoke (there is a reason that I write and don't sing). Naowarut Charoenca and Nipapun Kungskulniti of Mahidol University also read and helped edit early chapter drafts. In Germany, Martina Poetschke-Langer and Annette Bornhäuser provided crucial information and review. Eduardo Bianco provided in-depth assistance on the Uruguay chapter, and Adrianna Bianco of the Pan-American Health Organization graciously provided versions of her own case study of Uruguay to assist me in writing what is a relatively new story in tobacco control. I also want to thank Shaojun Ma of the China Medical Board and Gonghuan Yang of Peking Union Medical College for answering questions and reading drafts of the China chapter. I owe a very special thank-you to Yinqi "Mike" Zhang, who served as my primary research assistant and reference manager while I developed the book. This book also would not exist without the support of many individuals at Johns Hopkins University Press, especially Kelley Squazzo for believing in the project and Sara Cleary for her meticulous editing.

Finally, I must thank my husband, Ralph Wipfli, my parents, Don and Jan Schall, and my children, Ray, Ian, and Ana, for their unwavering support. It is not a simple task to write a book while working full time (including frequent international travel) and raising three small children. They make it possible for me to "have it all."

When I remember my paternal grandfather, I think of his anger and how the anger of millions upon millions of former smokers like him has been lost because they have not lived long enough to raise their voices. I believe it is my obligation to document his rage and the rage of his counterparts around the world. Although my grandfather never got to see me become the professional and mother that I am now, there is one thing I am certain of—that he would be proud of me and of all those who have worked to make the FCTC a reality.

ACS	American Cancer Society
AFTA	Asian Free Trade Agreement
ASEAN	Association of Southeast Asian Nations
ASH	Action on Smoking and Health
BAT	British American Tobacco
CDC	Centers for Disease Control and Prevention
COP	Conference of Parties
FAO	Food and Agricultural Organization
FCA	Framework Convention Alliance
FCTC	Framework Convention on Tobacco Control
FDA	Food and Drug Administration
GATS	Global Adult Tobacco Survey
GATT	General Agreement on Tariffs and Trade
GTCR	Global Tobacco Control Report
GYTS	Global Youth Tobacco Survey
IDRC	International Development Research Center
INB	Intergovernmental Negotiating Body
ITGA	International Tobacco Growers' Association
NGO	non-governmental organization
PMI	Philip Morris International
PSAC	Policy Strategy Advisory Committee
TFI	Tobacco Free Initiative
TIRC	Tobacco Industry Research Committee
UICC	Union for International Cancer Control
UN	United Nations
UNICEF	United Nations Children's Fund
WCTOH	World Conference on Tobacco or Health
WHA	World Health Assembly
WHO	World Health Organization
WTO	World Trade Organization

The Global War on Tobacco

CHAPTER ONE

A World Connected by Cigarettes and Disease

Our modern world is defined by connectivity. Today's communication tools spread information from the depths of the Amazon to the farthest reaches of Central Asia to New York City within seconds. Instant transnational communication is central to modern globalization defined by deepening global integration, which occurs as capital, goods, people, and ideas diffuse across national boundaries. Although communication and markets are global, regulation and norms are not. National regulations of industry, for example, can vary greatly in different parts of the world.[1] Even among industrialized countries as similar as Canada, the United States, and Germany, there are different social norms and expectations of government and the private sector.[2] These variations are often more pronounced among high-, middle-, and low-income countries. Systems of environmental regulation, for example, were not established in most middle-income countries until the 1990s, 20 years after high-income countries had implemented such laws.[3] Many low-income countries continue to lack basic environmental protections. Even where national regulations are in place, rule compliance differs between cultures and governments.[4] Governments, especially those in low-income countries, may lack the capacity and political will to implement and enforce existing regulations.

The lack of standard international regulations and norms has created ethical and practical dilemmas for multinational companies, governments, and international organizations, especially in providing and protecting global public goods. In the absence of either global or national regulations, multinational companies have occasionally ignored the industrial pollution that they generated, adopted a free-for-all attitude toward resource exploitation, and violated internationally accepted human rights.[5] A number of health-related events in the first decade of the twenty-first century illustrate the impact that regulatory approaches (or the lack thereof) in one country can have on the peace and security of another country, including the 2003 SARS outbreak, the H1N1 pandemic response, the continued spread of multi-drug-resistant tuberculosis, the 2008 melamine scandal in

China, and the growing threat of antibiotic resistance.[6,7] Consequently, there were urgent calls for global mechanisms capable of regulating transnational forces that affect population health, and innovative new governing approaches to address health at the global level emerged.[8–10]

The global tobacco epidemic provides one of the best illustrations of the challenges and opportunities that globalization presents to providing and protecting health within our fragmented international system. The successful transnational tobacco industry has used numerous elements of globalization, including trade liberalization, foreign direct investment, and global communications, to expand its markets to low- and middle-income countries where effective tobacco control programs are not in place. As a consequence, global health has been substantially diminished. Tobacco-related deaths, a completely manmade epidemic, have become the leading cause of preventable death in the world. Tobacco kills more people than HIV, malaria, and tuberculosis combined.[11] In 2013 alone, tobacco killed nearly six million people.[12] More than five million of those deaths resulted from direct tobacco use, whereas more than 600,000 were the result of non-smokers being exposed to secondhand smoke. Based on current trends, tobacco-related deaths are projected to reach eight million per year by 2030, with approximately 80% of those deaths forecasted to occur in low- and middle-income countries.[13] A shocking one billion people are projected to die from tobacco use this century, 900 million more than in the last.[14]

As the industry's global ambitions became clear and the evidence of a growing pandemic emerged, a committed group of individuals and organizations sought to challenge the tobacco industry's expansion and to control tobacco use. They used modern communication technologies and virtual networks to spread information, coordinate activities, and elicit responses from local, national, and international authorities. The global response included the first ever negotiation of a binding international law under the auspices of the World Health Organization (WHO), the WHO Framework Convention on Tobacco Control (FCTC). This book tells the FCTC story, from its start as an unlikely civil society proposal in the mid-1990s to its entry into force in 178 countries as of June 2014. In doing so, the book seeks to advance our understanding of how non-state actors and international institutionalization can impact global governance of health.

The term *global governance* emerged in international relations literature in the 1980s and became increasingly popular during the 1990s as the diffusion of power and authority and the realignment of significant actors—state and non-state, local and international, public and private—required an understanding of governance systems for which existing theories of international cooperation were clearly inadequate.[15] Broadly speaking, global governance refers to "the many ways individuals and institutions, public and private, manage their common affairs."[16] Global governance literature emphasizes the multiplicity and diversity of the actors involved in the management of international affairs and the influence of social networks.

The evolving global health environment of the first decade of the twenty-first century fit well into the theoretical global governance paradigm, and much has been written about emerging structures of global health governance.[17-19] Like other topics in global governance, global health governance literature focuses on the rise of actors involved in the management and delivery of health services around the world, the complexity of overlapping legal regimes pertaining to health (e.g., environment, labor, trade), and the innovative new public–private partnerships with novel decision-making structures (e.g., GAVI Alliance, The Global Fund to Fight AIDS, Tuberculosis and Malaria, and UNITAID). Although much of existing global health governance literature references the example of tobacco control and the emergence of the FCTC, to date there have been no in-depth accounts of the FCTC from its inception to its legally binding implementation. There is also surprisingly little analysis of the FCTC process in relation to the evolving nature of our international system and the role of international institutionalization in the formation of global norms and domestic policy.

As the first treaty negotiated under the auspices of WHO and the first collective response to non-communicable diseases (NCDs), the FCTC provides a critical case study for anyone interested in understanding how issues rise to global importance and whether, and through which mechanisms, developments at the international level can influence domestic policymaking and create standard regulations and norms within states. Much of the governance literature in international relations, for example, emphasizes bargaining and coercion between countries to explain global governance.[20] Alternatively, comparative politics literature has stressed how responses vary depending on local political and economic conditions.[21-23] These studies emphasize divergent policy choices when confronted with common problems or different ways to implement policies in similar cases.

Both international relations and comparative politics approaches fail to adequately explain the tobacco case. International relations approaches provide insight into the role of powerful states in governing the international system, but they discount the influence that smaller, lower-income states and civil society have on the international system. They also neglect the international policy and norm convergence that takes place in the absence of powerful external pressure.

In the case of tobacco, many countries chose to conform their domestic polices to international standards and agreed to the development of a formally binding instrument in the absence of external force. Moreover, small, lower-income countries and civil society were central in the FCTC's development, at times directly challenging the will of powerful high-income countries.

The specification of comparative political models is also called into question by growing empirical evidence showing that economic, environmental, and public health policies are growing more alike.[24–26] Tobacco products, prevalence of smoking, and the burden of disease caused by tobacco differ greatly among countries and regions. Accordingly, one would expect, a priori, to find significant variation in national choices and not the emergence of global policy convergence. Tobacco control, however, is defined by remarkable consistency among countries. Standard policy packages and communication campaigns are routinely translated and implanted in dramatically different contexts.

More recent, alternative explanations for the acceptance of international ideas, policies, and norms within countries have focused on cross-national communication and learning over time, or *diffusion*.[27–29] Diffusion occurs in the absence of formal or contractual obligation, or external pressure, and it is decentralized and unconnected in nature—such that the policies of one country can influence another's without the country of origin even knowing it. Initial research suggests that communication that results from international policy processes may create cross-national learning about a policy or norm and can gradually increase acceptance in reluctant countries, paving the way for the emergence, modification, and even ratification of international agreements. Consequently, efforts aimed at encouraging and facilitating international information sharing could be essential in enhancing global health governance. In other words, the process itself is the product.

Tobacco, and the FCTC in particular, illustrate the "governance by diffusion" approach. From the start of the FCTC process, diffusion arguments were made to justify the investment in the treaty negotiations. WHO officials claimed, for example, that the power of the FCTC was not the treaty itself, but that of the treaty-making process.[30] The negotiating process, they argued, would intensify international communication about tobacco, and the information shared would accelerate the passage of tobacco control policies throughout the world. Some claimed early on that the information shared through the negotiating sessions and at preparatory meetings was successfully leading to policy change. Even the senior vice president for corporate affairs at Philip Morris International advised an industry conference in 2003 that, regardless of the future of the FCTC, "the

Treaty [process] has had a significant influence on us, simply because it has accelerated the pace of regulation in individual countries."[31]

Indeed, in the early 1990s, few could imagine a world in which 178 countries
would agree to an international law requiring countries to implement domestic
tobacco control policies. However, by 2003, the 192 member states of WHO were
willing to unanimously adopt the FCTC, and the treaty became binding international law less than two years later. Within five years, more than 168 states had
signed the treaty and 154 states had ratified it, making it one of the most quickly
accepted treaties in UN history. FCTC-relevant policies were subsequently adopted worldwide. The policy progress achieved between 2007 and 2010 is forecasted to result in approximately 7.5 million fewer smoking-related deaths by
2050.[32]

This remarkable turnaround is worthy of further study. It is very much a story
focused on the role of communication and collaboration between non-state
actors and their ability to set agendas and elicit responses from states and international institutions. For decades, international networking and collaboration
between individual scientists and advocates supported the transfer of tobacco
control policies from one country to another. However, it was the ability of tobacco control advocates to access and influence WHO and other international
institutions in the mid-1990s that eventually led to the emergence of the FCTC.
The FCTC negotiations vaulted the tobacco control issue up political agendas
within countries and led to intense information sharing and, eventually, simultaneous adoption of tobacco control policies in numerous diverse countries. Additional philanthropic investment for international training, capacity building, and
collaboration, primarily carried out by non-governmental organizations, further
intensified policy diffusion, resulting in a completely revolutionized global tobacco control environment within a few short years.

The FCTC is a double-sided story. On the one hand, the FCTC is a singular
tale of an international effort to develop a new instrument in global health governance. On the other hand, the FCTC is made up of nearly 200 individual stories
about how new international legal norms were understood, negotiated, and
translated into domestic legislation. To capture this story, this book is divided
into two parts. The first part offers a global perspective on the processes and
players influencing the treaty's development and implementation. Chapter 2 focuses on the history of the tobacco industry's global expansion, the rise of evidence linking tobacco use to death and disease, and the process through which
initial international networking among a small handful of public health professionals evolved into a global movement committed to the idea of an international

legal regime for tobacco. Chapter 3 concentrates on the FCTC negotiations, its adoption by the World Health Assembly (WHA), and its entry into force. The chapter provides insight into the major debates, explores the influence of civil society and private industry, and analyzes the final textual outcomes. Chapter 4 reviews FCTC implementation in the decade following its adoption by the WHA. The chapter looks at the global institutionalization of the treaty regime, including the establishment of the Conference of Parties (COP) to the WHO FCTC, which has subsequently negotiated implementation guidelines for many articles in the treaty and launched negotiations of the FCTC's first protocol related to illicit trade in tobacco products—formally adopted at the fifth session of the COP in November 2012. The chapter also explores the contribution of significant philanthropic funding for FCTC-relevant capacity building and policy advocacy, and it evaluates major shifts in policies within countries. The chapter ends by considering some of the most significant transnational challenges facing the FCTC as it enters its second decade.

Part II of the book shifts away from the global perspective to focus on individual country experiences with tobacco control and the impact the FCTC has had on domestic policy decisions. Chapters 5–8 provide qualitative descriptions and analyses of how the FCTC intersected with political, economic, and legal forces influencing tobacco control in Thailand, Uruguay, Germany, and China. The country case studies selected in this book represent three of the four major categories of countries that participated in the FCTC. Thailand represents the handful of middle-income countries that had strong tobacco control laws going into the FCTC but looked to the treaty to help institutionalize its past tobacco control success and gain solidarity in its efforts to keep the transnational tobacco companies at bay. Uruguay represents the larger number of lower-income countries that had little domestic tobacco control prior to the launch of the FCTC and needed the FCTC as a foundation upon which to stand up to the forces that had successfully hindered tobacco control for decades. China and Germany represent countries that were home to large tobacco companies and that fought against a strong FCTC. Few expected these countries to use the treaty to move their tobacco control agendas forward domestically. I have left out the group of high-income countries that had already instituted comprehensive tobacco control programs domestically and that helped initiate the FCTC process (Canada, Australia, Norway), as their stories have been told elsewhere.

The countries selected are also diverse in relation to geography, economic development, government structure, tobacco use, tobacco industry presence, and social norms. The countries break down traditional divides between developed and developing countries often perpetuated in existing public health publications, as well as in literature focused on the transfer of norms and laws. The format of each case study roughly follows the same outline, starting with the tobacco control situation prior to the launch of the FCTC process, followed by a description of the country's involvement in the FCTC negotiations, and finally focusing on if and how the treaty has been used to advance tobacco control policy since FCTC ratification. The stories are distinctly different from one another and I have allowed them to evolve in different ways—reflected in slightly different structures in each case. The final chapter concludes with a summary of the main themes found throughout the book and their implications for global health and global governance given current trends and processes.

The global war on tobacco, and the FCTC process in particular, has broad implications for other areas of global health governance—especially those attempting to address public health problems defined by modern lifestyles, such as diet, physical inactivity, and alcohol. These factors underlie the emerging pandemics of NCDs: coronary heart disease, diabetes, cancer, and chronic lung disease. There has been increasing global policy attention paid to these risk factors and their consequent diseases, including the 2011 United Nations High Level Meeting on Prevention and Control of NCDs and multiple follow-up resolutions within WHO. Based on its experience developing, negotiating, and implementing the FCTC, the tobacco control community has much to offer the broader NCD policy movement. The FCTC itself represents a key weapon in the NCD battle, as tobacco remains one of the leading causes of NCDs globally.

To date, however, there has not been a serious effort to replicate the FCTC process in other areas of global health. Generally speaking, this is illustrative of the international community's shift away from its focus in the 1990s on international legal regimes to address global public goods toward non-binding public–private agreements during the past decade. This redirection is to some extent based on the notions that international legal processes in other areas failed to achieve their ultimate objectives and that non-binding mechanisms can be effective.[33]

In regard to the FCTC, much confusion remains over *how* the process worked, *whether* the process worked, and if it was *worth the investment* of time and money. As described in this book, the definition of success for the FCTC has constantly evolved, from whether countries could ever agree to a text, to what that text would include, to whether countries would ratify, to whether its entry into force would translate into domestic policy changes, to how many lives have been saved as a result of the FCTC's existence. As the bar has moved, the FCTC has continued to meet (at least minimum) expectations. If anything, the FCTC has proven itself to be an incredible tool for policy advocacy and advancement in many countries. However, as could be expected, implementation of the treaty is not even in all countries or regions, and the treaty faces significant challenges as it enters its second decade. By telling the global FCTC story and analyzing its impact on domestic politics, this book records what has worked and what hasn't and addresses the central issue of whether future investments in binding international legal processes are effective and appropriate in advancing global health.

PART ONE

THE GLOBAL TALE

CHAPTER TWO

One Hundred Years in the Making

The notion of the Framework Convention on Tobacco Control arose in the last decades of what can accurately be referred to as the "cigarette century."[1] It was during the first decades of the twentieth century that the structure of the modern tobacco industry was formed and its political influence was solidified. As the century wore on and the negative health consequences of active and passive smoking became undeniable, high-income countries began implementing policies to control and prevent tobacco use. Despite subsequent reductions in tobacco consumption in select countries, the global tobacco epidemic grew exponentially in the latter years of the twentieth century. The tobacco industry took full advantage of trade liberalization, foreign direct investment, new production technologies, global communications, and other elements of the emerging globalized economy to gain customers in low- and middle-income countries and to increase profits. It was in this context that tobacco control advocates began working together across borders, eventually calling for the development of an international legal instrument to rein in the increasingly transnational tobacco industry. Although much has already been written about the rise of tobacco use and efforts to control it in the United States and other high-income Western countries, it is still critical to briefly review the tobacco story over the past century to understand the zeitgeist that led to the FCTC negotiations and why so many countries were engaged in the process.

Establishment of the Industry

The modern tobacco industry was born out of the cigarette. Until the latter half of the 1800s, tobacco consumption was almost entirely confined to chewing, snuff, and pipe smoking by middle-aged men. Three major inventions led to the popular use of tobacco in the form of cigarettes. First was the discovery of a standard method for producing flue-cured tobacco leaves in Virginia in 1839. Flue-cured "yellow" tobacco resulted in a mild-flavored smoke more appealing to the general public than that of the harsh dark tobacco previously available. Second was the 1852 invention of safety matches, which made smoking easier. Third was James Bonsack's invention of the first practical cigarette-making machine in 1880, which significantly cut manufacturing costs.[2] In 1884, James Duke, a tobacco producer in North Carolina, formed a partnership with Bonsack. By the end of the year, Duke had produced 744 million cigarettes, more than the national total in 1883.[3] The cost savings associated with the Bonsack machine allowed Duke to sell his cigarettes for less than his competitors.

In 1890, following a series of price wars, Duke merged with several American competitors to form the American Tobacco Company. In an effort to resist a raid by Duke on the British industry, British companies joined together and formed Imperial Tobacco in 1901. In 1902, the American and British tobacco companies agreed to stay in their respective countries and united to form British American Tobacco (BAT) and sell both companies' brands abroad. As a result, the conglomerate controlled virtually all tobacco production and trade worldwide.[4]

The US Justice Department filed an anti-trust suit in 1907 against the American Tobacco Company, and in 1911 the company was formally broken into several major companies, including the American Tobacco Company, R. J. Reynolds, Liggett & Meyers Tobacco Company, Lorillard, and British American Tobacco. Although national tobacco monopolies in some countries limited the international markets of these major tobacco companies, they nevertheless were the dominant players in the global tobacco business throughout the twentieth century.

From the earliest days of their existence, modern tobacco companies have understood the importance of resisting governmental regulation and controls on tobacco. Although the deadly effects of tobacco were not well characterized until the 1950s, the effects of nicotine on the body were recognized much earlier. In 1890, tobacco appeared in *Pharmacopoeia*, an official US government listing of drugs.[5] However, the reference to tobacco was dropped before passage of the 1906 Food and Drug Act, the legislation that created the US Food and Drug Administration (FDA), when tobacco companies threatened that tobacco-growing states would not support the law as long as tobacco was included on the list of drugs to be regulated by the new agency. Consequently, tobacco fell into a regulatory vacuum, not defined as a food or a drug—a precedent that had global implications.

It was also at this time that the tobacco industry first tested revolutionary new advertising techniques and learned of the powerful influence that advertising had on its business. Even though the Bonsack machine produced cigarettes for a mass market, such a market did not exist at the turn of the twentieth century. To create demand, James Duke turned to new and highly effective marketing methods that set a precedent for the industry. In 1913, the newly independent R. J. Reynolds launched a massive, months-long campaign before introducing its Camel cigarettes. Theirs was the first modern cigarette campaign with national marketing and advertising; by 1923, Camel cigarettes controlled 43% of the US market.[6]

A main objective of many early cigarette advertising campaigns was to develop the tobacco market among women. In an effort to make smoking more socially acceptable for women, one marketing strategy for the tobacco industry was to link cigarette smoking to the liberation of women and the women's rights movement. In 1924, for example, Marlboro cigarettes were first launched as a cigarette for women. These campaigns were successful, and public acceptance and the prevalence of smoking grew.

The dramatic rise in demand for cigarettes resulting from these early advertising campaigns demonstrated that advertising could create demand for a product. Consumption is seen as an act of the imagination—that is, one buys not just the product but also the attributes the product is said to confer.[7] Consequently, tobacco industry advertising has used images of freedom, rebellion, health, fitness, stress relief, wealth, weight loss, and sex appeal to construct and perpetuate social attributes linked to cigarette smoking.

The Rise of Health Concerns and Scientific Evidence

By 1930 the tobacco industry was skilled in promoting its products to the mass public, and social acceptance of smoking grew. As a result, cigarette consumption rose dramatically. Between 1930 and 1940, per capita cigarette consumption in the United States doubled, and by 1939, 66% of men under the age of 40 smoked.[8] The rise in popular cigarette use was accompanied by worrying trends. By 1930, the United Kingdom had the highest rate of lung cancer in the world, rising five times faster than all other cancers, and by 1948, lung cancer had become the second most common type of cancer among men in the United Kingdom. Suspicions of a relationship between the two trends led to the first scientific studies linking cigarette smoking to lung cancer.

Scientists in Germany first began making statistical correlations between cancer and smoking in the 1930s.[9,10] In 1938, Dr. Raymond Pearl of Johns Hopkins University reported that smokers do not live as long as non-smokers.[11] Three key case-control studies, all linking smoking to a higher risk of lung cancer, were published in 1950.[12-14] In 1953, Ernst Wynder demonstrated that cigarette tar caused tumors on the backs of mice, and in the following year, Richard Doll and

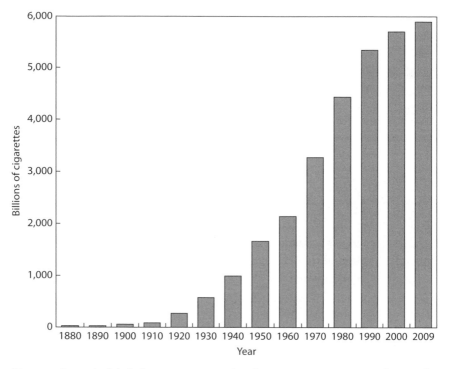

Figure 1. Annual global cigarette consumption from 1880 to 2009. Data from Eriksen M., J. Mackay, and H. Ross. *The Tobacco Atlas.* 4th ed. Atlanta, GA: American Cancer Society and New York, NY: World Lung Foundation, 2012

Bradford Hill published a nationwide prospective study of British doctors that found the risk of lung cancer greatly increased among smokers relative to the risk among comparable non-smokers.[15,16]

These early scientific studies and their potential impact on tobacco consumption provoked the tobacco industry, which created the Tobacco Industry Research Committee (TIRC) in 1954 to conduct its own scientific studies. On January 4, 1954, the TIRC released the "Frank Statement to Cigarette Smokers" in 448 newspapers throughout the United States. In it the industry declared: "We accept an interest in people's health as a basic responsibility, paramount to every other consideration in our business . . . We believe the products we make are not injurious to health . . . We always have and always will cooperate closely with those whose task it is to safeguard the public health."[17] At the same time, the industry began to mass-market filtered cigarettes and, later, low-tar formulations that promised a "healthier" smoke. The number of cigarettes with filters increased from 2% in

1950 to more than 50% in 1960. The strategy was effective and cigarette sales boomed.

For decades the tobacco industry continued to deny the relationship between cigarette smoking and disease and pointed to its own research as evidence that smoking was not harmful or addictive. As recently as 1994, the top seven tobacco industry executives swore under oath to the US Congress that they did not believe smoking to be addictive.[18] However, in 1998, as a condition of settling ongoing litigation with the attorney general of Minnesota, the tobacco industry was forced to make available confidential documents dating back to the early 1930s that proved the companies had been aware of the harmful effects of smoking since the mid-1950s and had implemented a strategy to hide this information to undermine the growing evidence base. The confidential industry documents detail how they used their own research institutes to produce contradictory results, paid scientists to challenge established scientific methods such as epidemiology, and publicly rejected claims that their products were dangerous or addictive.[19-21] This industry strategy was effective in perpetuating the impression among the public that the scientific community had not yet reached a consensus on there being a causal relationship between tobacco use and disease.

Despite the tobacco industry's efforts, growing scientific consensus regarding the link between smoking and cancer was reflected in the 1962 Royal College Report in the United Kingdom and the first Surgeon General's Report in the United States in 1964, both entitled "Smoking and Health."[22,23] The reports concluded that cigarette smoking is causally related to lung cancer, and they recommended legislative action to control its use. The compilation of data provided the critical rationale for legislative action to control tobacco use, including the initiation of health warnings on all cigarette packages and advertising restrictions on radio and television. In many ways, these reports signify the birth of modern tobacco control efforts.

Elsewhere in the world, this scientific consensus was also heard. For example, in 1963, the *South African Medical Journal* called on the South African government urgently to ban smoking in public places and on public transport, eliminate tobacco advertising, require health warnings, and increase taxation of cigarettes.[24] It would take decades, however, before even one of these recommendations was implemented in South Africa.

In 1964, US-based Philip Morris launched the most infamous of all cigarette ad campaigns—Marlboro Country. The campaign "Come to where the flavor is. Come to Marlboro Country" associated cigarettes with the American West and with a masculine approach to life that rejected concerns about the potential health risks associated with daily pleasures. The campaign transformed a stagnant American company into a transnational business phenomenon, and Marlboros became one of the quintessential global cigarette brands.[25]

Policy Innovation and Transfer

Shortly after the release of the 1964 Surgeon General's Report, the United States implemented the first health warnings on cigarette packages and began public education programs on the harms of smoking. Other countries quickly followed suit, including Finland, Norway, and Singapore. Early tobacco control strategies differed from country to country, reflecting their unique political, social, and economic situations. Singapore and Finland successfully instituted comprehensive national tobacco control legislation in the 1970s that included advertising bans, health warnings on all cigarette packages, indoor smoking prohibitions, and tobacco taxes. Norway passed a comprehensive national advertising ban in 1975, but it did not consistently increase tobacco taxes. Sweden focused on continually raising the price of cigarettes, as well as on public education campaigns. In the United States, aggressive national regulation was difficult due to the longstanding relationship between the federal government and the tobacco industry. Moreover, US federalism dictated that states were responsible for many relevant policies (e.g., smoke-free air policies). Advocates in the United States primarily combated the tobacco industry by focusing on state and local action.

Secondhand Smoke

A major shift in policy approaches to controlling tobacco occurred in the late 1980s with the rise of new evidence that secondhand tobacco smoke caused death and disease in non-smokers. Until the late 1980s, the tobacco control movement was driven by scientific evidence linking active smoking to disease. Accordingly, the debate surrounding tobacco control often focused on smoker's rights. This changed after scientific evidence confirmed that a smoker's smoke harmed not only the smoker but also other individuals exposed to the smoke. The debate instantly shifted from the "right to smoke" to the "right to clean air."

Evidence of the negative health effects of secondhand smoke on the children of smokers was first published in the 1960s; major studies from Japan[26] and Greece[27] on lung cancer in adults appeared in 1981. Hirayama's study from Japan showed that wives of smokers were twice as likely to die of lung cancer as were wives of non-smokers. The industry attempted to subvert these early findings.

Following the publication of Hirayama's report, the *British Medical Journal* was flooded with letters to the editor claiming that the study was flawed by misclassification and confounding and statistical error.

Scientific consensus that passive smoking causes lung cancer in adults solidified in 1986 when the US Surgeon General, the International Agency for Research on Cancer, and the US National Academy of Sciences all concluded that secondhand smoke caused cancer in nonsmokers.[28] These reports were followed by a 1992 report by the US Environmental Protection Agency (EPA), as well as by the International Agency for Research on Cancer's updated 2002 report and the 2006 US Surgeon General's Report.

The tobacco industry extensively criticized the science used to link secondhand smoke to disease and attempted to provoke controversy over the health effects of secondhand smoke, the extent of exposures, and the effectiveness and costs of controlling it. Industry documents now reveal that as early as the 1970s the industry was aware that policies restricting or ending smoking in public places would severely undermine the social acceptability of smoking, create an environment that would make it easier for smokers to stop smoking, and discourage young people from starting.[29] Consequently, the industry aggressively fought national and regional clean indoor air measures throughout the world, often working through surrogates with undisclosed links to the tobacco industry, such as "hospitality associations." In Latin America, for example, Philip Morris and British American Tobacco, working through the US law firm Covington & Burling, developed the "Latin Project" to counter regulations aimed at creating smoke-free workplaces and public places.[30,31]

The consolidation of scientific evidence and the shift toward the protection of non-smokers led to a major new legislative agenda for tobacco control. Initially, actions were taken to separate smokers and non-smokers within the same space (non-smoking sections), followed by the creation of separate smoking spaces (smoking rooms), and then complete bans on indoor smoking. The movement toward complete bans was largely motivated by evidence that ventilation and air cleaning could not remove cigarette smoke toxins from the air.[32]

In 2002, Delaware became the first state in the United States to become completely smoke free in all public places and workplaces, including restaurants and bars. Other states followed suit, including New York in 2003, Massachusetts in 2004, Washington and Rhode Island in 2005, and New Jersey, Colorado, Hawaii, and Ohio in 2006. Canada's Northwest Territories passed a comprehensive smoke-free law in 2004. Also in 2004, Ireland, Norway, and New Zealand became the first countries to enact comprehensive smoke-free indoor air laws. In 2006, Uruguay became the first South American country to implement a 100% smoke-free regulation in workplaces, restaurants, and bars. Mauritius became the first country in Africa to adopt a comprehensive smoke-free law in November 2008.

International Communication

The rapid spread of smoking bans was just one result of increasing communication and networking among tobacco control advocates within and across countries. The first World Conference on Tobacco or Health (WCTOH) took place in 1967, and in 1970, the WHO adopted its first resolution on tobacco. Prior to the 1990s, however, international communication regarding tobacco control was largely limited to advocates in Western Europe and the United States. Scandinavian countries in particular in the 1970s were actively sharing information as well as different policies and programs. Even within the context of the World Health Organization, tobacco control was viewed as a policy area of concern exclusively to high-income countries.

This disparity began to change in the late 1980s when tobacco control professionals began to communicate more with colleagues in select middle-income countries. The communication was initially driven by the realization that the increasing international activity of the major tobacco companies was setting the stage for a global public health crisis. Between 1970 and 1998 the tobacco industry underwent a complete transformation and globalization. Prior to the 1980s, large tobacco companies mainly exported cigarettes from facilities in the United States and Western Europe. In the last few decades of the twentieth century, however, the bulk of tobacco production moved to low- and middle-income countries. Production grew by 128% between 1975 and 1998 in these countries, while falling by 31% in high-income countries.[33] Land in the United States devoted to tobacco growing was halved, whereas it was almost doubled in China, Malawi, and the Republic of Tanzania.[34]

In 1998, 75% of the world's cigarette market was controlled by just four companies: Philip Morris, British American Tobacco, Japan Tobacco, and the China National Tobacco Corporation.[35] The last's share was attributed almost entirely to its near monopoly in the enormous Chinese market, but the others were tireless in their pursuit of worldwide sales. The major transnational tobacco companies established a presence in almost every country. By the late 1990s, each of the three largest transnational tobacco companies owned or leased manufacturing facilities in more than 50 countries.[36]

Three main factors fueled the industry's global expansion and consolidation:

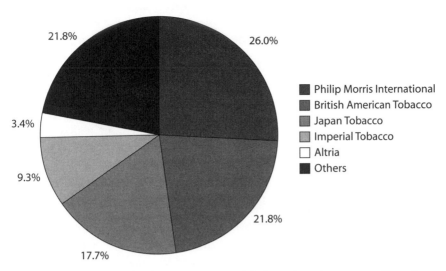

Figure 2. Transnational tobacco company global market share, 2011. Data from Credit Suisse, http://seekingalpha.com/article/299041-tobacco-stocks-defensive-play -in-uncertain-times

the opening of previously closed economies in the former Soviet Union, Eastern Europe, and China; the pressure exerted on countries by the World Bank and the International Monetary Fund to liberalize foreign investment laws and privatize state-owned tobacco companies; and the expansion of free trade areas in Asia and Latin America.[37] By the late 1990s, smoking prevalence rates among men in many low- and middle-income countries exceeded 60%.[38] Whereas female smokers were previously uncommon, industry penetration and marketing resulted in increased prevalence, especially among young women.[39] As highlighted by these globalization trends, smoking prevalence and the burden of disease, regardless of income level, were growing increasingly similar.

Recognizing these trends, key individuals such as Richard Peto, a professor of medical science and epidemiology at the University of Oxford, and Greg Connolly of the Massachusetts Department of Health reached out to potential colleagues in targeted middle-income countries in an effort to prompt tobacco control. Thailand's tobacco control efforts are explored in depth in the second part of this book. Another principal example is Poland. The production and sale of cigarettes, which had been entirely controlled by the government, was one of the first economic sectors to be privatized in post-communist Poland. Within a few years, Polish tobacco companies were taken over by the transnational tobacco industry, and by the end of the 1990s, more than 90% of the country's tobacco industry belonged to transnational companies.[40] During this period of rapid privatization, government authorities made considerable concessions to the transnational tobacco companies, such as agreeing to keep tobacco taxes low throughout the first half of the 1990s. As a result, in the early 1990s the average price of a pack of cigarettes in Poland was lower than the price of a loaf of bread.[41]

The transnational companies also started a lobby to promote their interests. An important part of their efforts involved establishing good relations with the emerging class of politicians, particularly economic and financial specialists. For example, the tobacco lobby made a donation to Lech Wałęsa, then leader of the Solidarity movement and an infamous chain smoker, in the hope of gaining his support.[42] One of the first goals of the tobacco lobby was to overturn the traditional ban on tobacco advertising. Although they were unable to roll back internal regulations against tobacco advertising on national television, they did manage to overcome restrictions in all other media, including public radio and the press, the first media to be privatized.

Subsequently, the tobacco companies introduced advertising techniques that Poles had never before experienced. Cigarettes quickly became the most heavily advertised product in the country. Toward the end of the 1990s, the transnational tobacco industry was spending $100 million per year on advertising cigarettes in Poland.[43] The use of state-of-the-art marketing techniques had a powerful effect on the previously unexposed Polish public. The number and percentage of occasional smokers rose, and the number of children experimenting with cigarettes, especially girls between the ages of 11 and 15, increased dramatically.[44]

In the midst of this transition, Dr. Witold Zatoński, a medical doctor at the Maria Skłodowska-Curie Memorial Cancer Centre and Institute of Oncology in Warsaw, was working with multiple international colleagues to counteract the industry. Richard Peto visited Poland and presented evidence to policymakers there showing that Polish life expectancy was no longer comparable to that of the Germans, their neighbors to the West, as it had been in the mid-1960s, but rather to the life expectancy of people in India and China.[45] This international comparison had a profound effect on the policymakers, who were unaware of the toll tobacco was taking on the Polish population. Zatoński worked with other international public health experts during this period, including Mike Pertschuk of the Advocacy Institute in Washington, DC, and Greg Connolly to challenge the industry's evidence and support tobacco control activities.[46] Working closely with Zatoński, these experts helped to sway public opinions about tobacco use and convince Polish policymakers to pass comprehensive tobacco control in 1995.

Global Communication

Despite the strong international collaborations that existed in Poland and a handful of other countries, international information sharing and learning was not easy in the late 1980s and early 1990s; in fact, the process was often long and tedious. The internet transformed international communication about tobacco control. Before the internet, for example, the tobacco industry could send its "experts"—often without disclosing their relationship to the tobacco industry—into a country, state, or locality to accomplish their political or public relations mission (e.g., arguing that secondhand smoke is not dangerous or that ventilation was a reasonable and feasible solution to the problems created by secondhand smoke). The "experts" would leave before any of the local public health advocates realized who they were. With the internet, it was suddenly possible for public health activists to rapidly learn who the international experts were and whether they had connections to the industry.

South Africa provided one of the first illustrations of the role internet networking could play in tobacco control. Following the dramatic political changes brought about by the end of the apartheid regime in the early 1990s, new political support emerged for the development of tobacco control legislation. In response, the tobacco industry significantly increased its lobbying activities in the country by sponsoring media workshops, lobbying the hospitality sector, creating front groups to oppose potential tobacco control measures, and reaching out to lawmakers. South African public health officials turned to international tobacco control experts for information and advice to prepare for the legislative process that lay ahead. Reflecting on one of the first preparatory meetings to discuss proposed legislation adjourned by the minister of health, a South African public health official recalled "I'm pretty sure they [the tobacco industry representatives] thought they were coming into a developing country where the knowledge base about the tobacco industry's behavior was poor. But we [public health officials] had been fully briefed—through our links with international colleagues—on everybody who was going to be before us. We knew all their arguments and that they could be countered easily."[47]

During this early period of international communication and policy transfer, policy makers in low- and middle-income countries often needed to be convinced that tobacco control was in fact an issue of concern. Domestic evidence was often required to move the policy debate forward, and intense collaboration and ongoing commitment from a small handful of dedicated individuals in and

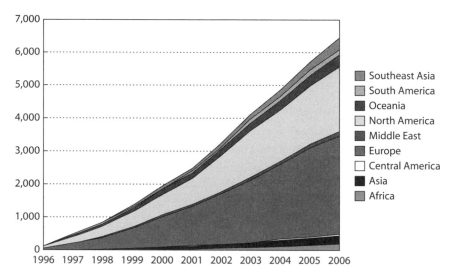

Figure 3. Membership in GLOBALink by geographic region, 1996–2006. Data from GLOBALink

outside the countries was required if there was to be any hope for the adoption of tobacco control policies.

By the mid-1990s, a small number of individuals from middle-income countries, including Poland, Thailand, and South Africa, were successful in pushing through tobacco control policies based on experiences in, and technical assistance from, high-income countries. As news of these developments began to spread, more and more individuals in low- and middle-income countries began turning to tobacco control experts from high-income countries with successful tobacco control programs for advice and technical assistance.[48–51]

Initial and haphazard tobacco control networking over the internet received a major boost in 1992 when the American Cancer Society turned over control of GLOBALink (then mainly a domestic US online tobacco control network) to the Union for International Cancer Control (UICC). The network's homepage contained news bulletins, electronic conferences, live interactive chat, and full-text databases (including news, legislation, and directories).[52] The internet was an inexpensive mechanism to distribute information anywhere in the world and link advocates, and membership in GLOBALink rapidly increased during the late 1990s to include a number of individuals from middle-income countries. In 1997, GLOBALink received the Tobacco or Health Award from WHO for its unique ability to bring together advocates for tobacco control policy.[53]

Globalization of Tobacco Control

As the twentieth century neared its end, many high-income countries and a handful of middle-income countries had made significant progress in reducing tobacco consumption. For example, in the 1960s, 50% of the US adult male population smoked, and by 1970, nearly 75% of Polish men smoked.[54,55] In 2003, thanks to aggressive tobacco control programs, smoking prevalence decreased to 25% and approximately 40% among US and Polish men, respectively.[56] Between 1985 and 2000, lung cancer deaths in men decreased in many European countries: the United Kingdom (–38%), Finland (–36%), the Netherlands (–29%), Luxembourg (–24%), Austria (–23%), and Ireland (–22%).[57]

Global Presence of the Transnational Tobacco Industry

By the late 1990s, social, economic, and political globalization was having an ever-greater impact on national tobacco control efforts. Cross-border advertising, for example, was reducing the effectiveness of longstanding advertising bans. The industry's global presence was stronger than ever. By the mid-1990s, the Marlboro Man was one of the most widely recognized advertising symbols in the world, and he was declared the number one advertising icon of the twentieth century by *Advertising Age* magazine.[58] Marlboro comprised the greatest share of the global cigarette market, and Marlboro cigarettes could be found anywhere in the world. In the United States and Europe it was the only brand that continued to gain market share. Industry marketing of Marlboro and other international brands increasingly tapped into globalization trends to develop a "global mental framework" in association with manufactured cigarettes that helped the industry overcome markets that had thus far resisted the industry's onslaught—a strategy employed to associate cigarettes with modernity, prosperity, and internationalism.[59,60] In India, for example, where traditional bidis and chewing tobacco remain the preferred forms of tobacco use, the industry used global brands such as Marlboro to encourage young smokers to switch to manufactured cigarettes.[61]

The industry also used well-funded and sophisticated corporate lobbying to resist regulation of their products throughout the world.[62] This lobbying effort was undertaken by the companies and third parties, targeted governments, international institutions, and the media.[63,64] In the Middle East, for example, the major transnational tobacco companies operating in the region formed the Middle East Working Group (MEWG), which later became the Middle East Tobacco Association (META), to promote and defend the interests of the companies in the region.[65] Companies enlisted prominent political figures to provide information and lobby for them, including an Egyptian member of parliament, a former assistant secretary general of the Arab League, and even, at one point, the secretary general of the Gulf Cooperation Council of Health Ministers, who was also the Kuwaiti undersecretary for health.[66]

In Africa, the industry developed the International Tobacco Growers' Association (ITGA) to lobby on its behalf. The ITGA, along with other international consortiums such as the International Council on Smoking Issues (ICOSI), later known as the International Tobacco Information Centre (INFOTAB), targeted the Food and Agricultural Organization (FAO) of the United Nations and WHO in particular.[67]

The US Congress also remained a vital lobbying target. During the first half of 1998, the industry reportedly spent more than $43 million on lobbying against federal tobacco legislation sponsored by Senator John McCain. The industry's advertising campaign against the bill was, according to Kathleen Hall Jamieson, the Dean of Communications at the University of Pennsylvania, the highest amount ever spent on a sustained issue advocacy campaign in the United States.[68]

It was in this environment that it became increasingly clear to tobacco control advocates that simply exporting the national experiences of high-income countries to partners in low- and middle-income countries was not enough to counter the unregulated global tobacco industry. Despite many individual successes, domestic tobacco control groups recognized the need for multinational cooperation and effective international action to control transnational factors.

The Rise and Institutionalization of the Framework Convention Approach

Between 1970 and 1998 the World Health Assembly (WHA), the decision-making body of the World Health Organization, adopted 17 resolutions on different aspects of tobacco control.[69] Although nations occasionally referenced these resolutions when passing national tobacco control legislation, the lack of any legally binding authority made the resolutions inconsequential for many nations. A new approach was needed.

The idea of using WHO's constitutional authority to establish an international legal regime for tobacco control can be traced back to a report prepared by the WHO Expert Committee on Smoking Control in 1979.[70] The report suggested using the organization's treaty-making power granted in its constitution to develop binding obligations if other non-binding resolutions on tobacco did not produce results in a reasonable time. WHO's constitution mandates the organization and its member states to work for the "the attainment by all peoples of the highest possible level of health."[71] The constitution, approved on April 7, 1948, includes article 19, which grants extensive powers to the WHA to prepare and adopt standards, legislation, conventions, and agreements to protect and promote international public health. Never in its first 50 years of existence did WHO utilize this treaty-making power, though, in part because it was mainly staffed by medical doctors and scientists who traditionally focused on technical, clinical approaches to disease prevention and control.

A decade after the 1979 Expert Committee on Smoking Control report, Professor V. S. Mihajlov of the former Soviet Socialist Republics published an article on the feasibility of an international law for tobacco control.[72] Professor Mihajlov concluded that although it was "unrealistic at the present time, and indeed even ridiculous," he was convinced that the day would come when international health law would address alcohol and tobacco and their "enormous damage to health."[73] Shortly thereafter, the idea of developing an international treaty on tobacco control was crystallized through the work of two women: Ruth Roemer and Allyn Taylor.

Ruth Roemer was a public health lawyer based at the University of California, Los Angeles, who had been commissioned by WHO to write a book on the use of legislation to tackle the world tobacco epidemic in the early 1980s.[74] A decade later, Roemer was impressed by an article written by a Columbia law student, Allyn Taylor, who advocated for WHO to utilize its (until then) neglected constitutional powers to develop a legal framework to advance global public health.[75] Roemer contacted Taylor to suggest that such a legal framework could be used for tobacco control.[76]

During the next few years Taylor focused her dissertation work on the development of international treaty law for tobacco control, while Roemer campaigned for the idea at various international public health conferences and engaged with senior staff at WHO to promote the convention approach. Roemer gained a number of prominent allies through her efforts, including Judith Mackay, a long-time challenger of the tobacco industry in Asia and an influential WHO consultant. Derek Yach, then chairperson of the 1993 All Africa Tobacco Control Conference, also became a critical supporter of the treaty idea at this time.

In 1994, at the Ninth World Conference on Tobacco or Health in Paris, Roemer, Taylor, and Mackay drafted, introduced, and successfully passed a resolution calling on national governments, ministers of health, and WHO to "immediately initiate action to prepare and achieve an International Convention on Tobacco

Control to be adopted by the United Nations."[77] The conference marked the first international forum in which the idea of a FCTC was formally endorsed and was the beginning of official efforts to secure support from within WHO.

The director of the WHO tobacco control unit, Neil Collishaw, was a member of the WCTOH Resolutions Committee. After the 1994 conference he worked with other tobacco control advocates to include the mandate to develop an international framework convention for tobacco control in WHO's official policies. Collishaw, who had joined WHO from Health Canada, also worked closely with Canadian tobacco control advocates to reach out to members of the Canadian delegation to the 1995 WHA and ask them to formally propose support for the idea. Canadian delegate Jean Lariviere drafted an official resolution requesting that the director general of WHO report on the feasibility of developing an international instrument for tobacco control. Lariviere also worked with delegates from Finland, Mexico, and Tanzania to build support.[78] Consequently, Lariviere's draft text was adopted by the executive board (EB95.R9) and later by the WHA (WHA48.11).[79]

Roemer and Taylor were subsequently commissioned by Collishaw to write a background paper setting out various options for developing an international legal strategy. Their paper recommended the development and implementation of a framework convention approach.[80] The WHO director general produced a brief report for the 1996 WHO executive board that summarized the key recommendations of the background paper. Because Canadian officials were not part of the executive board in 1996, Lariviere worked closely with Kimmo Leppo of Finland and John Hurley of Ireland to propose and pass the 1996 resolution of the executive board, which called for the development of a WHO FCTC and related protocols (EB97.R8).[81] A few months later, the WHA adopted the resolution (WHA 49.17), formally institutionalizing the idea of the FCTC within WHO.[82]

Although the 1996 resolution established the official mandate to initiate a *conversation* about the FCTC, there remained extensive opposition within the WHO secretariat and executive board to using article 19 to draft and adopt a treaty on tobacco control. WHO's legal counsel, in particular, was resistant to the idea of negotiating the treaty under the auspices of WHO. Only a year earlier, they had written a letter to Roemer claiming the proposal was ambitious to a fault.[83] It was not until two years later and the election of Dr. Gro Harlem Brundtland as WHO director general in 1998 that WHO become serious in its intentions to make the FCTC a reality.

The role of Brundtland as the champion of the FCTC cannot be overstated. Brundtland held a strong personal commitment to tobacco control and the FCTC in particular from the very start of her administration. This commitment was in part due to her experience with tobacco control in the 1980s in Norway and in part the result of aggressive lobbying by a handful of her closest advisors. Tobacco control leaders Richard Peto, Judith Mackay, and Derek Yach were members of Brundtland's transition team and were responsible for advising her in the development of her strategic plan. They were able to take advantage of their position and a unique moment in history to convince Brundtland that it was the right time to push the FCTC forward. From the beginning, Brundtland was committed to having a special cabinet project on malaria, but invited other specialties to make pitches for a second special focus. Judith Mackay, Richard Peto, and Neil Collishaw put forward the idea of tobacco. There were many reasons why tobacco was attractive to Brundtland.[84] First, after years of dysfunction, WHO desperately needed strong, clear, and innovative leadership. Second, momentum for tobacco control was strong after the conclusion in the United States of the Tobacco Master Settlement Agreement and the release of the previously confidential tobacco industry documents.[85] Third, the health consequences, burden of disease, and economic evidence supporting tobacco control was available to justify global attention to the issue. In the years preceding the election of Brundtland, the Canadian government, through its International Development Research Center (IDRC), had supported extensive research on the economics of tobacco control in low- and middle-income countries. This evidence would become critical as the treaty progressed.

Although these three factors alone would probably not have been enough to convince many incoming WHO directors to take on the FCTC, Brundtland was different. Although she was trained as a medical doctor, she had had a long, successful political career. As former prime minister of Norway, as well as the former minister of environmental affairs and commissioner of the Sustainable Development Commission for the UN secretary general in the 1980s, Brundtland had experience negotiating treaties, was comfortable leading the member states through a highly political process, and knew how to get things done in the UN system. She was also prepared to stand up to the transnational tobacco companies following her experience confronting oil companies who were drilling in the North Sea after the Ekofisk oil spill disaster.[86,87] The pieces of the puzzle had suddenly come together to take tobacco control, WHO, and global health governance in a dramatically new direction.

Tobacco Free Initiative

When Brundtland was elected director general at the 1998 WHA, she immediately established the Tobacco Free Initiative (TFI) as a special cabinet project. She appointed Derek Yach as its founding director and ordered regional directors to institute corresponding TFI teams in each of WHO's regional offices. Derek would lead TFI for the following four years, after which he was promoted to assistant director general of non-communicable disease and mental health. Dr. Vera Luiza da Costa e Silva took over TFI in 2001 and led the department through 2005, at which time the FCTC was binding international law.

TFI's mission was to establish global leadership in four priority areas: (1) global information management, (2) development of nationally and locally grounded action, (3) establishment of strong and effective partnerships, and (4) global regulation and legal instruments (i.e., leadership of the FCTC). In addition to funding from the WHO regular budget, significant funding for TFI's work was provided by the United Nations Foundation/United Nations Fund for International Partnerships. Smaller contributions were made by individual governments and private sector companies to support specific TFI activities.

Derek Yach appointed a highly dynamic team to work with him at WHO headquarters. Chitra Subramaniam was appointed director of communications and media. Famous for her investigation of the Bofors-India Howitzer deal, which is widely believed to have contributed to the electoral defeat of former Prime Minister Rajiv Gandhi in 1989, Subramaniam was a vigorous advocate who was not afraid to ruffle feathers. Another key member was Douglas Bettcher, a technical wizard with a diverse multidisciplinary background in international relations, public health, and medicine. Bettcher was put in charge of legal and procedural issues relating to the development of the FCTC. He dedicated himself entirely to the task and remains a major force behind the FCTC to this day. A team of young technical and administrative assistants (author included) also worked tirelessly to quickly move WHO's global tobacco control agenda forward in the early days of Brundtland's term.

The dynamism of TFI at the time stood in stark contrast to many of WHO's other technical divisions, and it quickly gained a reputation for breaking traditional norms and expectations in the organization. In addition to the TFI team at WHO headquarters, regional TFI teams carried out activities on their own and in partnership with each other. As the FCTC process evolved, the regional teams would become core focal points for coordination and action among countries in their respective regions.

Media and Advocacy Campaigns

Under Subramaniam's direction, media and advocacy campaigns funded by the UN Foundation were quickly launched to inform governments and civil society of the urgent need for a coordinated global response to tobacco. The media campaign sought to move tobacco control issues to the top of national and international political agendas and to the center of national public health debates. The campaign, entitled "Don't be Duped—Tobacco Kills," was launched in San Francisco in November 1999 and initially targeted 16 priority countries. With the campaign, WHO sought to change the tobacco control debate from human fragility to corporate accountability. The campaign was aggressive in publicizing the dangers associated with tobacco and sought to counter the global marketing practices of the tobacco industry that lure customers, especially young people, through sponsorships, advertising, and glamorization of tobacco in film, music, and sports. In doing so, the campaign sought a new language and a new direction for tobacco control. In contrast to the traditional No Smoking sign, the campaign coopted the tobacco industry's use of images, music, fun, and freedom to advance their public health agenda. The symbol of the 1999 campaign was two Marlboro-esque cowboys riding into the sunset with the caption, "Bob, I've Got Cancer." In the 2001 campaign, a similar image was used but one of the horses was missing its rider and the caption read, "Secondhand Smoke Kills," implying that the other cowboy had been killed by the pictured cowboy's secondhand smoke.

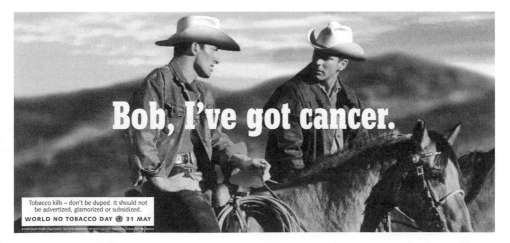

Figure 4. WHO poster for World No Tobacco Day, May 31, 2000. World Health Organization

An advocacy campaign entitled "Channeling the Outrage" engaged and supported nationally based social entrepreneurs and change agents from the media,
non-governmental organization (NGO) community, health professionals, and
the private sector in target countries. Change agents were selected based on their
demonstrated interest in tobacco control, access to their own networks, and ability to influence policy in their areas of focus. The participants from Zimbabwe,
for example, worked on agricultural diversification, whereas in Thailand they focused on point-of-sale advertising. In India, the emphasis was on the bidi industry, and individuals in Germany and Ukraine targeted the power of the tobacco
industry.

Once selected, change agents were sent for advocacy and media training with
Stanton Glantz at the University of California, San Francisco, and Mike Pertschuk
at the Advocacy Institute in Washington, DC. The program proved effective at
influencing tobacco control efforts in the participating countries. The work of
Martina Poetschke-Langer, the change agent in Germany, is explored in the German case study presented in chapter 7.

In addition to the campaign's focus on individual change agents, TFI's program also focused on building institutional advocacy capacity within member
states. A major portion of the funds provided by the United Nations Foundation/
United Nations Fund for International Partnerships was channeled into capacity-
building grants for NGOs. In 1999, WHO awarded the British-based Action on
Smoking and Health (ASH) a grant to identify how to involve civil society in the
FCTC negotiations. With the help of the internet and GLOBALink, ASH was able
to mobilize a loose network of NGOs around the world, which evolved into the
Framework Convention Alliance (FCA) by 2000.

Multi-sectoral Collaboration

Beside its support for civil society, TFI also established numerous global partnerships and initiated global multi-sectoral cooperation among international organizations with a stake in tobacco control. TFI initiated a Policy Strategy Advisory
Committee (PSAC) to gain policy coherence on tobacco control, solidify support
for WHO activities, and expand the base of advocacy and action. The PSAC included representatives from the World Bank, the United Nations Children's Fund
(UNICEF), the World Self-Medication Industry (WSMI, which represents pharmaceutical companies who produce nicotine replacement therapy to help smokers
quit), the International Nongovernmental Coalition Against Tobacco (INGCAT),
the Campaign for Tobacco-Free Kids, and the US Centers for Disease Control and

Prevention (CDC). The PSAC was mandated to guide and support TFI in its mission. Generally speaking, the development of the PSAC accomplished the goal of bringing the various tobacco control players together. However, there was occasional conflict and stress between TFI and PSAC members once the FCTC negotiations began, and TFI had to work at balancing its role as technical resource, advocate, and legal secretariat. The PSAC was eventually dissolved in 2001.

In addition to the PSAC, WHO advocated for the establishment of an Ad Hoc Interagency Task Force on Tobacco Control and, in 1999, the UN secretary general asked WHO to convene the task force.[88] The creation of the task force resituated the focus of UN tobacco policy from the UN Conference on Trade and Development and, in doing so, shifted the tobacco debate in the UN to address health first and supply second. Fifteen UN organizations, as well as the World Bank, the International Monetary Fund, and the World Trade Organization participated in the task force.[89]

The task force provided a mechanism for partnerships with agencies in sectors other than health and resulted in collaborative projects with the FAO, the International Labor Organization (ILO), UNICEF, and the World Bank. The World Bank's 1999 publication, "Curbing the Epidemic" provided perhaps the single most important tool in preparation for the FCTC negotiations. The report identified cost-effective interventions to enhance revenues and promote health.[90] Based on numerous economic studies conducted by researchers at the World Bank and others (many supported by the IDRC), the report encourages governments to adopt a multi-pronged strategy that is tailored to the conditions within their respective countries. In particular, the World Bank found that demand-reduction strategies, such as tax increases, promotion bans, warning labels, restrictions on public smoking, and widened access to nicotine replacement therapies and other cessation therapies were the most effective strategies in the short term.

The World Bank report provided a credible evidence base for global tobacco regulation and helped to reverse the longstanding perception that the tobacco industry was too economically beneficial to developing and tobacco-producing countries to allow for effective regulation. The report emphasized the need to primarily focus on demand-reduction strategies as opposed to supply reduction, arguing that population growth alone would continue to fuel tobacco product demand despite successful efforts to reduce overall prevalence and consumption. This argument was particularly popular in countries that wished to address tobacco use but didn't want to upset the population of their tobacco-producing areas. The impact of the report was greatly increased by a $500,000 grant from the CDC for its global dissemination.

Global Information Management

A core objective of TFI was to develop a global information system to manage and track global tobacco use and control efforts. In December 1998, TFI convened a meeting in Geneva with the CDC, UNICEF, the World Bank, and representatives from countries in each of the six WHO regions to discuss the need for standardized mechanisms to collect tobacco use information on a global scale. The outcome of this meeting was the development by WHO and CDC of a Global Tobacco Surveillance System.

The first data collection mechanism developed for the system was the Global Youth Tobacco Survey (GYTS). The GYTS is a school-based survey designed to enhance the capacity of countries to monitor tobacco use among youth and to guide the implementation and evaluation of tobacco prevention and control programs. The GYTS uses a standard methodology for constructing the sampling frame, selecting schools and classes, preparing questionnaires, following consistent field procedures, and using consistent data management procedures for data processing and analysis.

Within a decade, TFI and CDC used GYTS to survey more than two million students from 11,000 schools in 150 countries. The data collected became a fundamental source of information about the current global tobacco epidemic, and it forecast changes occurring in tobacco use among young people. Significant findings included similar cigarette smoking rates between girls and boys in many countries, early initiation of tobacco use worldwide (smokers were 11 years old on average), widespread exposure to secondhand smoke in public places, and high demand for smoking cessation assistance.

Other instruments in the Global Tobacco Surveillance System include the Global Health Professions Student Survey, which monitors tobacco use and behavior among future healthcare providers; the Global School Professional Survey, which collects data from teachers and administrators from the same schools that participate in the GYTS; and, eventually, the Global Adult Tobacco Survey (GATS), a household survey that monitors tobacco use among adults. GYTS and GATS would evolve into core instruments used to monitor the effectiveness of FCTC implementation in countries and are explored in more depth in the next chapter.

Litigation and the Industry

Between 1950 and 1998, the tobacco industry enjoyed a successful record in civil litigation that was unique to almost any industry. The industry never paid one cent in settlements or awards for any injuries claimed by cigarette smokers in their civil lawsuits. However, in the early to mid-1990s, more than 40 states commenced litigation against the tobacco industry, seeking monetary, equitable, and injunctive relief under various consumer protection and anti-trust laws. Faced with the prospect of defending multiple actions nationwide, the four major US tobacco companies (Philip Morris USA, R. J. Reynolds, Brown & Williamson Tobacco Corporation, and Lorillard Tobacco Company) sought a congressional remedy, primarily in the form of a national legislative settlement. In June 1997, the National Association of Attorneys General and the tobacco companies jointly petitioned Congress for a global resolution that would include FDA authority over tobacco. Senator John McCain of Arizona carried the bill. However, in the spring of 1998 Congress rejected both the proposed settlement and an alternative proposal submitted by McCain. The tobacco industry launched the costliest lobbying campaign in the history of the US Congress against the bill, despite their initial participation in its development.

While the proposed legislation was being discussed in Congress, some individual states began settling their litigation against the tobacco industry. On July 2, 1997, Mississippi became the first state to reach a settlement. During the next year, Florida, Texas, and Minnesota followed, with the four states recovering a total of more than $35 billion. The settlement with the state of Minnesota was unprecedented in terms of monetary relief, injunctive requirements, and the aforementioned release of approximately 35 million pages of internal industry documents.[91] In November 1998, the attorneys general of the remaining 46 states, as well as of the District of Columbia, Puerto Rico, and the Virgin Islands, entered into the Tobacco Master Settlement Agreement, which forced the four major US tobacco companies to pay $264 billion over a period of 25 years to compensate for tobacco-related health costs.[83]

Key to these settlements and turnaround in litigation was the release of the previously confidential industry documents. The documents revealed that the industry knew for more than four decades that smoking tobacco caused cancer, that they were aware of the addictive nature of nicotine, and that they manipulated nicotine content to increase addiction. The documents also outlined a well-developed and well-executed strategy to cover up this information, target vulnerable populations, including youth and women, and undermine tobacco control efforts.

TFI was quick to recognize the potential these preliminary victories in US courts created for litigation in other countries. Members of the legal team from the Minnesota case were pulled in as technical experts, helping to prepare reports, technical briefings, and consultations. In 2000, TFI partnered with the government of India to host the International Conference on Tobacco Control Law in New Delhi, through which several recommendations were issued to facilitate international litigation.[92] During the next year, litigation was launched in more than a dozen countries, ranging from personal class-action litigation to healthcare recovery and public interest petitions. Cases were also launched in Canada and the European Union (EU) that accused the tobacco companies of smuggling and requested financial compensation for lost revenue and injunctive relief to prevent future smuggling.

TFI also recognized the potential power of the industry documents to move its own agenda forward. In 1999, Brundtland established a committee of experts, chaired by Thomas Zeltner, director of the Swiss Federal Office of Public Health, to investigate the possibility of tobacco industry interference in WHO's work on tobacco. The committee's detailed report documented the industry's many attempts to prevent, delay, and weaken WHO tobacco control activities. The industry staged events to divert attention away from the public health issues raised by tobacco use, attempted to reduce budgets for scientific and policy activities carried out by WHO, pit other UN agencies against WHO, distorted the results of scientific studies on tobacco (including those carried out by the International Agency for Research on Cancer), worked to discredit WHO as an institution through third-party critics, and used surrogates to influence WHO decisions.

The release of the WHO inquiry corresponded with the release of *The Insider*, a film starring Russell Crowe that told the story of tobacco industry whistle blower Jeffrey Wigand. The film was a box office hit in 1999 and exemplified the social and political awareness of the tobacco industry's despicable behavior at the time and a growing willingness to take action against it in courts and through policy. This social and political atmosphere facilitated TFI's work and provided a supportive atmosphere in which to launch the FCTC negotiation process.

CHAPTER THREE

Those Who Want and Those Who Do Not . . .
The FCTC Negotiations

Before getting into the story of the Framework Convention on Tobacco Control negotiations, it's important to understand what a framework convention is and what the FCTC was originally intended to do. International conventions, including framework conventions, are treaties: written agreements between states that are governed by international law. Treaties are often referred to by different names, including agreements, conventions, covenants, protocols, and exchanges of notes. The 1969 Vienna Convention on the Law of Treaties contains the basic principles of treaty law, the procedures for how treaties become binding and enter into force, the consequences of a breach of treaty, and principles for interpreting treaties.[1]

The basic principle underlying the law of treaties is *pacta sunt servanda,* which means that every treaty in force is binding for the parties to it and must be performed by them in good faith. The other important principle is that treaties are binding only for states that have agreed to be governed by the treaty; they are not binding for third-party states without their consent.

The term *framework convention* does not have a special legal meaning in international law, but it is generally used to describe international agreements whose principle function is to establish a system of governance and a basic institutional structure around a specific issue.[2] Framework conventions are commonly followed by more specific commitments and institutional arrangements in the form of protocols. Protocols are subsequent treaties that follow a similar process of negotiation, adoption, and ratification as the initial framework treaty. In addition to protocols, a treaty's governing body can also make interim decisions in the form of guidelines, which are subsequent agreements regarding the interpretation of the treaty or the application of its provisions. Although guidelines are not independent treaties like protocols, and the language of guidelines may not always be mandatory, guidelines do provide general obligations for participatory states, and specific provisions of guidelines can induce mandatory action.

Framework conventions can vary considerably, as can their implementation.

Some conventions contain more detailed obligations and institutional mechanisms than others. Perhaps the best known framework convention is the United Nations Framework Convention on Climate Change, which includes reporting requirements, advisory bodies on science and implementation, and a financial fund to support treaty-related projects.[3] The UN Framework Convention on Climate Change was followed by the Kyoto Protocol, which commits its parties to internationally binding emission reduction targets.[4]

Generally speaking, framework conventions include:

- a statement of the convention's overall objective and guiding principles;
- basic obligations, including commitments to take national measures to address the relevant problem, to exchange information, to cooperate in scientific research, and to submit periodic reports;
- institutions, including a regular conference of the parties and secretariat (at a minimum), and possibly a scientific advisory body, implementation body, and financial mechanisms;
- processes by which to review implementation, promote compliance, and resolve disputes; and
- a law-making process for the adoption of more specific commitments, usually in the form of protocols and guidelines.

As traditional instruments of international law, framework conventions are agreed to solely by sovereign states through formal governmental approval.[5] The entry-into-force provisions of framework conventions usually specify a number of states that must ratify a treaty before it can become binding law. The required number of states varies between 20 and 50. Whereas a low number may speed up entry into force, a higher number will guarantee the convention's credibility.

In international law, the framework convention/protocol approach is typically used when there is no consensus for strong substantive measures, scientific understanding is evolving, and the problem being addressed is changing. The rationale for the framework convention is that it will help form cognitive and political consensus around an issue, and that it will provide states with a system of governance that allows them to proceed incrementally through guidelines and separate protocols.

Although the scientific evidence base for the harmful effects of tobacco was well established long before the FCTC negotiations, the World Health Organization nonetheless viewed the FCTC as necessary to promote acceptance of this evidence by its member states.[6] There remained great uncertainty at the time, especially within the WHO secretariat, about the member states' ability to find consensus on the harmful effects of tobacco, much less on specific tobacco control policies. The ever-changing landscape of the global tobacco industry also made the framework convention approach appealing.

Throughout history, international law has consisted primarily of rules and principles of general application that deal with the conduct of states and of international organizations in their relations with one another and, more recently, with private individuals, minority groups, and transnational companies. A key aspect of international law has been sovereignty, which gives states the exclusive right to exercise supreme political authority over a defined territory and people within that territory. The term *sovereignty* is closely associated with the concept of *political independence,* that is, allowing states to carry out their own domestic policies without external interference. Consequently, international law has primarily dealt with issues that have clear transnational applications.

In 1998, Dr. Gro Harlem Brundtland, the director general of WHO, applied this traditional understanding of international law when arguing for the FCTC. She reasoned that an international response was needed to address key aspects of tobacco control "that cross national boundaries." The framework convention, she said, "will seek to address key areas of [transnational] tobacco control such as: harmonization of taxes on tobacco products, smuggling, tax-free tobacco products, advertising and sponsorship, international trade, packaging and labeling, and agricultural diversification."[7]

Similarly, tobacco control advocates who promoted the idea of the FCTC pointed to the inability of individual states to control aspects of their domestic tobacco control environment without international collaboration. They pointed specifically to the negative impact of transnational advertising through satellite television and the internet, illicit trade encouraged by international price differentials, and decreasing prices caused by the inclusion of tobacco products in global and regional free trade agreements. Thus, the original rationale for developing the FCTC was not to develop a tool to assist countries in their domestic tobacco control efforts, but to reduce the negative effects of transnational forces and globalization on existing and future domestic policies and programs.

That being said, it was argued early on within WHO that the negotiation process would likely have an impact on domestic policies regardless of the final treaty outcome.[8] This argument was in part driven by ongoing doubts within the organization as to whether member states would accept a binding treaty text, something that had never been attempted before in the history of WHO. To justify the investment in the FCTC negotiations, members of the Tobacco Free Initiative (TFI) stressed potential supplementary benefits of the process, including domestic policy advancement in areas of tobacco control that had no cross-border impact, such as indoor smoking bans. In many ways, what was understood initially as a positive externality from the treaty-making process would arguably become its most valuable outcome.

Technical Working Group

At the fifty-second World Health Assembly in May 1999, resolution WHA52.18 established a technical working group to prepare proposed draft elements of the FCTC and an Intergovernmental Negotiating Body (INB) to draft and negotiate the proposed framework convention and related protocols.[9] The FCTC working group met twice as it developed its technical report for the WHA. The working group was chaired by Dr. Kimmo Leppo (Finland) and Dr. Margaret Chan (China; future WHO director general), and Dr. Vera Luiza da Costa e Silva (Brazil; TFI director, 2001–2005) served as the co-chair.

Luk Joossens, a tobacco control professional from Belgium, was asked to prepare the technical background paper for the working group meetings.[10] His task, and the task of the working group in general, was not to worry about the political process of adopting a convention, but to consider the scientific evidence base and to make recommendations as to what provisions a tobacco control convention should include. Like Joossens, the working group was decidedly pro–public health, with most country delegations still composed almost entirely of health officials. Although they were not particularly versed in treaty making, the working group decided not to simply recommend topics in report format, but, with help from WHO, to produce a provisional draft text of the treaty. The group also agreed not to cut proposals out of their draft treaty based on political realities, but instead to include all credible textual recommendations. Their final draft detailed the specifics of debate between various recommendations put forward by member states.

Within the working group, vigorous disagreement arose over how strong the framework convention should be;[11] their final draft concluded that "a majority of delegations favored a strong but general convention so that as many member states of WHO as possible could accede to it."[12] It stressed that the focus should be on "broad, comprehensive and inclusive principles, giving countries the necessary flexibility," although it was acknowledged that some delegates found it premature to identify specific obligations in the treaty.[13] The more compromising text, friendly to supporters of a weaker treaty, was likely composed by WHO staff who worried (and continued to worry throughout the process) that if progressive countries were successful in getting strong commitments into the treaty text, few member states would subsequently ratify it and, consequently, the credibility of WHO itself could be jeopardized.

In May 2000, the fifty-third WHA considered the working group's final report and called on the INB to begin negotiations on the text of the treaty.[14] At its first session, the INB accepted the working group's proposed draft elements of the FCTC as the base text from which to initiate negotiations. The acceptance of the text as a starting point had significant and lasting implications on the negotiations. First, it meant that a number of potentially deal-breaking issues were resolved before formal negotiations even began. For example, there was initial concern that some low-income, tobacco-producing countries would not participate in the process, or worse, that they might fight against the treaty due to fears that they would bear the consequences of supply reduction strategies and reduced demand for tobacco (i.e., direct employment losses), but gain few of the benefits because their populations already had low smoking rates.[15] By explicitly citing empirical evidence from the World Bank report,[16] which supported a primary focus on demand reduction strategies, the working group's draft treaty largely resolved this issue before the negotiations even began.

A second benefit of using the working group draft was the inclusion of strong public health language in the preamble, objectives, and guiding principles. Thus, from the beginning of the negotiations, there was the normative understanding that reducing the number of deaths and disease related to tobacco was the supreme objective. Finally, instead of having to build a strong treaty from the ground up, the negotiators could focus on taking out text where consensus was lacking. In areas of the treaty where there was little opposition, strong public health language endured.

FCTC Public Hearings

Immediately before the first INB session, WHO convened a public hearing on issues related to the proposed framework convention. Nearly all stakeholders in tobacco control, including the public health community and most of the major tobacco multinationals and state-owned companies, provided written and oral testimonies. More than 500 written submissions were received, and representatives of 144 organizations testified at the hearing. The testimonies were made available to the INB participants and to the general public.[17]

The hearing brought diverse organizations working on tobacco control together in one venue, thus providing an opportunity to galvanize societal interest in the FCTC. Widespread press coverage of the event also increased public awareness and support for the process. Jeffrey Wigand, the tobacco industry whistle blower who had become a household name after the release of *The Insider,* attended the hearing and provided a statement calling for strong regulation of the industry.

Testimonies during the two-day hearing reflected the priorities of the stakeholders present and foreshadowed the core debates that arose in the forthcoming treaty negotiations. Numerous public health groups, for example, spoke passionately about the major health concerns linked to passive smoking and argued that, to reduce tobacco-related death and disease, the FCTC must include obligations to reduce exposure to tobacco smoke.[18] Although prohibition of smoking in indoor public places was included as an option under article 8 of the working group's draft text, it was somewhat controversial at the time, even among tobacco control groups. It was difficult to argue the transnational dimension of secondhand smoke given that indoor smoking has little to no consequence for neighboring countries. The extent to which there was political motivation for indoor smoking bans (now an acceptable norm) was highly questionable in many regions, including Europe, and some public health groups feared that pushing for comprehensive domestic bans would appear extreme. However, the public health community's insistence that the FCTC retain language addressing secondhand smoke, framing it as a human rights issue, foreshadowed the eventual domestic content of the treaty.

Even more informative than the testimonies of the public health community were the positions shared by representatives of the tobacco industry, especially because the public hearing was the only official FCTC-related event in which the industry was welcomed to participate. The industry representative from Philip Morris, for example, admitted for the first time in an international forum that secondhand smoke is harmful.[19] Other company representatives, although not as forthcoming about secondhand smoke, did concede to the hazardous nature of active smoking.[20] The hearing also marked the first time that the strong divides between the companies in regard to their approach to the FCTC were evident. Philip Morris took a conciliatory tone, calling for partnership and collaboration in developing the FCTC into an effective tool for youth smoking prevention. Conversely, British American Tobacco (BAT) argued that the treaty approach was fundamentally flawed given the diversity of cultural, sectoral, and geographic interests with a stake in the future of tobacco. BAT also said that governments needed to be "free to develop the most appropriate policies for specific circumstances of their country."[21] Japan Tobacco International (JTI) disagreed with the fundamental objective of the convention: to reduce tobacco consumption. Representatives from JTI used the words *sovereign* or *sovereignty* 11 times and *appropriate* eight times in a five-minute speech at the hearing to emphasize the importance of government autonomy.[22] They contended that governments should be free to decide the nature of tobacco control regulations in their own context and should not be forced to implement one set of standards such as those embodied in the FCTC.[23] The tobacco companies largely sustained these positions over time as the negotiation process moved forward.

Intergovernmental Negotiating Body and Related Events

Between October 2000 and May 2003, the INB held six negotiation sessions. Each session lasted between one and two weeks. More than 170 member states participated in at least one of the negotiating sessions. The intensive process, which included numerous regional and technical consultations held in between the formal INB sessions, raised the political profile of tobacco as a global public health concern and increased awareness of effective interventions among policymakers. The high stakes associated with the prospect of binding obligations forced policymakers to study the issue carefully. The formal negotiating process also provided an ongoing forum for information sharing and learning among WHO member states. Many countries formed interministerial committees to establish their official governmental negotiating positions, thereby supplying the first opportunity for non-health sectors, including foreign affairs, finance, commerce, trade, and justice to jointly address tobacco issues. Some countries, particularly high-income countries, sent large delegations with at least one representative from each sector to the INB sessions.

TABLE 1
Timeline of Meetings by the Intergovernmental Negotiating Body (INB)
of the WHO Framework Convention on Tobacco Control

Meeting	Date	Location	No. of States Attending	No. of Country Delegates
INB1	October 16–21, 2000	Geneva	149	510
INB2	April 30–May 5, 2001	Geneva	157	548
INB3	November 22–28, 2001	Geneva	168	606
INB4	March 18–23, 2002	Geneva	160	585
INB5	October 14–25, 2002	Geneva	165	643
INB6	February 17–28, 2003	Geneva	171	699

The Overall Process

The WHO secretariat, led by TFI, administered the negotiations. Douglas Bettcher (future TFI director and WHO director of prevention of non-communicable diseases) was the TFI point person for the preparation of technical and legal documents provided to the INB. In addition to producing the official legal negotiating documents in which they were *supposedly* neutral, TFI also provided several capacity-building guides, such as *Building Blocks for Tobacco Control: A Handbook*,[24] and policy recommendations for numerous tobacco control issues that were disseminated throughout the process.

The secretariat worked closely with the INB chair and bureau, comprised of vice-chairs from each region, to prepare the necessary materials throughout the six INB sessions (INB1–6). The INB chair was an influential position throughout the process, ensuring that the complex, and at times contentious, negotiations continued to progress. The first chair, elected at INB1, was Celso Amorim, Brazil's permanent secretary to the United Nations. Amorim was the former Brazilian minister of foreign affairs and a skilled negotiator. Following his appointment to the United Nations he would be reappointed minister of foreign affairs and subsequently minister of defense in Brazil. Amorim presided over INBs 1–3 and was succeeded by Ambassador Luiz Felipe de Seixas Corrêa, also of Brazil, who saw the negotiations to conclusion.

Notably, neither chair was oriented in public health at the start of his term. Amorim was a tobacco smoker at the time. There is an infamous story of how, during a networking dinner before Amorim's election as chair, Brundtland proposed that chairing the negotiations would provide a good opportunity for him to quit smoking. Amorim's wife responded positively to the proposal, insisting that he take on the role and quit. He did both.

The choice of Brazilian officials to chair the negotiations was highly strategic. Not only were both ambassadors skilled diplomats, but Brazil was simultaneously a major tobacco producer and a world leader in tobacco control. Brazil's chairmanship of the negotiations helped to create a political bridge between countries that were tobacco producers and those that were not, and it exemplified the compatibility between producing tobacco and controlling tobacco use. Reflecting on his time as chair, Amorim highlighted the challenge of preparing a treaty that would bring countries together and, most importantly, would be ratified by them afterward. "The starting point," he recalled, had to be "the common will to impose limits on the consumption of tobacco."[25]

Negotiators decided at the end of INB1 that the discussions would proceed in three simultaneous working groups. Thus, at INB2 (Geneva, April 30–May 5, 2001) three concurrent working groups divided the responsibility of drafting the proposed elements of the convention. Working group 1, chaired by France and Thailand, addressed technical issues within the treaty, including tobacco product disclosures, youth access, packaging and labeling, treatment of tobacco dependence, exposure to tobacco smoke, tobacco product content regulations, and advertising, promotion, and sponsorship. Working group 2, chaired by Canada and Zimbabwe, addressed surveillance, information exchange, tobacco taxes, tax-free and duty-free sales, subsidies, illicit trade, and agricultural substitution. Working group 3, chaired by New Zealand and Egypt, addressed logistical and implementation issues, including the treaty's institutional framework, settlement of disputes, liability and compensation, final clauses, financial mechanisms, and cooperation in the scientific, technical, and legal fields.

The early negotiations were tedious, contentious, and often confusing. The chair's draft released in January 2001 was a largely unreadable mess of overlapping proposals. No one knew quite how to manage the intense and divided participation of so many member states. Between INB4 and INB5, a revised chair's text was prepared that clarified the variety of proposals resulting from the active participation of member states in the first four INBs. At the first reading of the new chair's text at INB5, six priorities were identified for discussion by open-ended, informal drafting groups: (1) advertising, promotion, and sponsorship; (2) financial resources; (3) illicit trade in tobacco products; (4) liability and compensation; (5) packaging and labeling; and (6) trade and health. Other informal drafting groups dealt with legal, institutional, and procedural issues and use of terms. Members of INB5 subsequently went to work focusing the negotiations.

Based on the output of these working groups, Ambassador de Seixas Corrêa issued a revised chair's text on January 15, 2003, for negotiation at the sixth and final INB (February 17–28, 2003). Major stumbling blocks remained concerning trade and health, advertising and sponsorship, financial resources, and the reservation clause (which allowed countries to ratify the convention but elect to be bound only by specific provisions of their choosing). As the end of the session neared, it was clear that the delegates needed more time to resolve a number of key issues. When consensus had not been reached on the final day of the session, the plenary body agreed to hold one final meeting at midnight. Despite the late hour and exhausting two weeks beforehand, the commitment to find consensus was evident. The plenary room was full of delegates in the early morning of February 28, and at 4 AM, they agreed to transmit the final text of the FCTC to the fifty-sixth WHA and requested that the chair draft a resolution recommending adoption by the member states.[26]

Negotiating Blocks

The speed at which the FCTC was negotiated should not be mistaken for a lack of rigorous debate. The negotiations were marked by intense disagreement between countries on a number of key issues, including advertising and sponsorship bans, youth access, packaging and labeling, financial assistance, and trade and health. Although country positions shifted according to the issues at hand, there were clear negotiating blocks. As Chair Amorim described, there were "those who have done; those who want to do; those who want to but cannot; and those who do not want to do."[27]

"Those who have done" was a dedicated group of high-income countries who had instituted strong tobacco control policies domestically and had played a key role in initiating the FCTC process. Throughout the negotiations they fought for the inclusion of strong measures in the FCTC. These countries, including Australia, Canada, Finland, Norway, and New Zealand, often championed the public health proposals emanating from the non-governmental organizations, and they partnered closely with smaller and lower-income countries to increase their influence. They also provided strong examples of domestic tobacco control success and worked with NGOs and TFI to disseminate evidence concerning effective tobacco control approaches and to build capacity among low- and middle-income country delegations.

"Those who want to do" was a handful of middle-income countries who were in the process of implementing new tobacco control programs and who looked to the FCTC to help further institutionalize tobacco control. These countries, including South Africa, Thailand, Brazil, and Poland, partnered with the previously described high-income countries to argue for a strong FCTC. They had extensive expertise and experience in tobacco control and took on key leadership roles in the process, including within the bureau and committees. They also formed important regional alliances with other low- and middle-income countries.

In contrast, Amorim's third group—"those who want to but cannot"—included many African, English-speaking Caribbean, and Pacific Island countries who had little or no experience with tobacco control and lacked the capacity to develop or implement effective tobacco control policies and programs. As the negotiations progressed, these countries united in their arguments for social justice and public health, joining the other two negotiating blocks in arguing for a strong FCTC. As described by Muyunda Ililonga, executive secretary of the Zambia Consumer Association, "There was a collective realization by the African countries' delegates that tobacco was, after all, not benefiting the economies of the poor African countries, while at the same time the tobacco industry was increasingly focusing on Africa for their future market."[28] Delegations from low- and middle-income countries comprised the majority of the INB, and by uniting together, they greatly increased their influence on the process.

Finally, a small group of high-income states—"those who do not want to do"—who were home to the transnational tobacco companies, fought against strong commitments in the FCTC and, at times, threatened to derail the entire process.[29] These countries became known as the "Big Four": Japan, home to and part owner of JTI; Germany, then home to Rothmans, the fourth largest transnational tobacco company at the time; the United States, home to Philip Morris; and China, itself the owner of the China National Tobacco Company. Each of these countries faced significant criticism for their positions throughout the process, although the United States received by far the greatest condemnation, in part due to the heavy presence of US-based NGOs at the negotiations. Tobacco companies are powerful in the United States because of strong national lobbying efforts and generous campaign contributions, particularly to the Republican Party. At the start of the FCTC process, however, there was still hope that the United States would be a productive participant in the negotiations. This enthusiasm quickly extinguished when the Clinton administration was replaced in 2001 by that of George W. Bush, who received significant financial support from the tobacco industry in the 2000 US elections.

Once President Bush took office, the United States objected to, among other things, provisions that warning labels on cigarette packages be printed in the main language(s) of the country of sale, the precedence of public health over trade, and a comprehensive ban on advertising.[30] The position of the United States was strikingly close to that of Philip Morris. It sought to eliminate, for example, 10 of the 11 provisions that Philip Morris wanted deleted in the text. Mirroring tobacco industry arguments, the United States cited constitutional and free trade concerns as reasons for opposing provisions on advertising and trade. The United States' position was so extreme that its senior public health official and head of the US delegation, Tom Novotny, resigned in May 2001.

The David versus Goliath nature of the negotiations became a rallying point for many low- and middle-income countries that previously may not have been inclined to work together. One avenue they used to overcome the influence and pressure of the Big Four was the formation of regional negotiating blocs. At the first African intersessional meeting in Johannesburg, South Africa, in March 2001, the African negotiators were able to find so much common ground that they made the decision to negotiate with a single voice. Working together, the African countries provided a powerful counterforce to the influential high-income countries that were attempting to weaken the treaty, and they were able to dramatically change the direction of the negotiations. Other regional groups decided to follow suit, including the WHO Regional Office for South-East Asia (SEARO), the Association of Southeast Asian Nations (ASEAN), and the WHO Regional Office for the Western Pacific (WPRO). Even the European Regional Office, in cooperation with host countries, facilitated coordination in subregional groups and held a region-wide coordination meeting before the last round of negotiations in early 2003. The regional alliances particularly helped low-income countries (e.g., the Pacific Islands and the English-speaking Caribbean), which could not afford to send large delegations to Geneva or cope with the demands of the protracted and simultaneous negotiating sessions.[31]

Regional consensus gained through intersessional negotiating meetings facilitated the development and adoption of the FCTC, especially in the later stages of the negotiations. Not everyone was pleased with the emergence of the regional groupings. Gregory Jacob, a member of the US delegation and a scathing critic of the FCTC process, has argued that WHO's regional structure encouraged a split between high-income and middle- and low-income countries.[32] In reality, regional blocks encouraged low- and middle-income countries to stand up and not back down to the comparatively isolated US position regarding the treaty. Consequently, the existence of the regional blocks did slow down progress because countries occasionally chose to stick to their regional positions instead of compromising individually. This stubbornness, however, is likely to have facilitated a stronger final treaty text.

Civil Society Participation

Representatives of civil society were key participants throughout the negotiations, although their involvement was often an issue of contention, and their access fluctuated throughout the process. During INB1, countries agreed to adhere to existing WHO rules, which only allowed NGOs in formal relations with WHO to attend and make statements at the conclusion of plenary sessions and at the discretion of the chair. Technically, these rules meant that official participation was limited to a small handful of NGOs, and these NGOs became the official links between the INBs and extensive civil society networks. Whereas NGOs were initially required to submit prewritten statements to the secretariat and were only invited to read them by the chair at the end of a plenary session if time permitted, after a while the process relaxed and NGOs became more integrated, making spontaneous statements at the invitation of the chair.

Also at INB1, Canada and Thailand successfully led an effort to ensure that participating NGOs had broad access to the process, including observation of breakout meetings (i.e., regional meetings). However, following efforts led by the United States and China, NGOs were denied access to informal breakout groups in the final stages of the negotiations (INB6), frustrating many of the NGO representatives who had grown accustomed to access.

Two global networks of NGOs coordinated FCTC lobbying efforts worldwide: the Framework Convention Alliance (FCA), a group of more than 200 organizations in 93 countries, and the Network for Accountability of Tobacco Transnationals (NATT), a group of more than 75 organizations in 50 countries. Although neither network had official relations with WHO, founding members of the networks did (e.g., the American Cancer Society and the Union for International Cancer Control with the FCA, and INFACT [now known as Corporate Accountability International] with NATT). These NGOs used their access to send large delegations of diverse individuals to push for a strong FCTC.

There was much overlap in the membership and activities of the FCA and the NATT. Both networks were known for impressive cooperation and collaboration across borders by NGOs in high-, middle-, and low-income countries, which was mostly facilitated through e-mail communication and was driven by a common interest in reining in a rogue industry. The ability of these diverse NGOs to find policy consensus on specific issues provided a strong message of preferred solutions to participating countries. For example, all groups eventually agreed on the need for a complete ban on indoor smoking in public places. Their unity on the issue shifted delegate perceptions in relation to secondhand smoke.

Because NGOs were not formal participants in the FCTC negotiations, they adopted strategies and tactics from other treaty-making processes to influence national delegations. NGOs kept a "death clock" running, for example, which tallied the number of people killed by tobacco worldwide since the beginning of negotiations and underlined the urgency of the situation. Activists also dressed up in "Mr. Butts" costumes to deliver petition signatures in favor of a strong FCTC to country delegates, and they displayed banners that depicted the many victims of tobacco around the world.

One particularly effective action by the FCA was the daily publication of the

Alliance Bulletin. The *Bulletin*, first published during INB1, served educational and informational purposes for the delegates, and it effectively put pressure on pro-tobacco countries. The FCA produced the *Bulletin* each night of the negotiations in French, Spanish, and English, and delivered it to delegates in the morning. The Bulletin included reports on the previous day's events and contained technical information about the topics under consideration that day. Given the INB structure, with multiple concurrent sessions occurring at any one time, the *Bulletin* acted as an informative daily newspaper.

Although the *Alliance Bulletin* did serve as an important source of news and information for many delegates, it became notorious for its inclusion, on its back page, of the Orchid and Dirty Ashtray Awards for countries involved in the treaty negotiations. These seemingly insignificant notes on the back of the *Bulletin* became important labels as the negotiations continued. The first thing that delegates arriving at the Geneva Convention Center did in the morning was obtain a copy of the *Bulletin* and flip it over to see who won the infamous awards. Some governments took the awards seriously—at least the Dirty Ashtray Award. Wanting to be seen as responsible contributors to the process despite their opposition to a number of core provisions, Chinese delegates complained to the FCA and even raised the topic during the plenary session when it won two Dirty Ashtray Awards during INB6.[33] The Japanese delegation received six Dirty Ashtray Awards, the most of any country.[34] However, the FCA crowned the United States the overall winner, awarding it five Dirty Ashtray Awards and a Special Lifetime Achievement Award during INB6—a testament to how frustrated the FCA was with the US position on key provisions.[35]

Throughout the FCTC negotiations, the United States was subject to intense criticism from the FCA, the NATT, its domestic tobacco control community (many of whom were members of the FCA), and members of the US Congress. Members of civil society were concerned from the beginning that the treaty's power could be severely undermined by US opposition. The American Cancer Society, the American Heart Association, the American Lung Association, and the Campaign for Tobacco Free Kids (all FCA members) called on the United States to stop undermining efforts to reduce death and disease caused by tobacco around the world. In a published letter to President Bush, Congressman Henry Waxman (Democrat, California) said, "the position of the US has been in virtual lockstep with the tobacco industry throughout the treaty negotiation."[36]

As the negotiations were ending, with no sign of the United States, Germany, or Japan retreating from their obstructionist roles, NGOs switched from a "shape up" to a "ship out" message, calling on these delegations to remove themselves

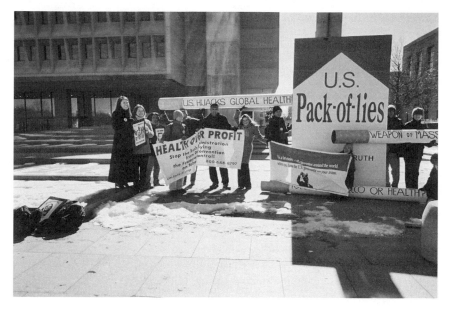

Figure 5. Demonstration in front of the US Department of Health and Human Services, February 12, 2013. Essential Action

from the negotiations altogether. The NGOs launched e-mail, fax, and telephone campaigns targeting the head of the US delegation, Kenneth Bernard. Leading up to the final round of negotiations, advocates held a demonstration in front of the US Department of Health and Human Services that featured a 10-foot-high pack of Marlboro cigarettes labeled "US Pack of Lies," complete with gigantic cigarettes bearing phrases like "US Fronts for Big Tobacco," "US Hijacks Global Health," "Weapon of Mass Destruction," and "Tommy T: Tobacco or Health?" The slogans touched on the double standard between the US government's rhetoric about protecting the world from terrorism and its inaction in controlling the deadly tobacco industry.

During the final FCTC negotiating round, NGOs lined up in front of the plenary room where the final draft was being deliberated and held signs calling for the US delegates to go home. According to Hatai Chitanondh, a Thai delegate who worked closely with NGOs throughout the negotiations, this action had an immediately noticeable effect: "Every time I had proposed the wordings for health over trade from the second negotiating round up to that moment, the U.S. delegate would come up and rebut me strongly. But that time, they kept their mouth shut, choosing to have [a small group of other tobacco-friendly nations] confront me instead."[37] In targeting the United States, NGOs also effectively isolated Japan and Germany.

In addition to confronting the Big Four and acting as the conscience of the negotiations, NGOs served as an ongoing tobacco control university.[38] Throughout each INB session, NGOs partnered with TFI and individual states to hold lunch seminars and workshops on various technical aspects of the convention. They also published a number of capacity-building guides and policy recommendations, which were distributed to delegates with the aim of strengthening national tobacco control programs. Through these briefings, NGO representatives directly lobbied country delegates, particularly those from low- and middle-income countries. They submitted amendments to texts, held face-to-face meetings in corridors, and distributed position papers.

There is no question that NGOs greatly influenced the outcome of the FCTC negotiations. The contribution of civil society to the FCTC was officially recognized when member states incorporated article 4, guiding principle 7 into the text of the FCTC, which reads, "The participation of civil society is essential in achieving the objective of the Convention and its protocols."[39] However, some have questioned whether the NGOS helped or hurt the FCTC process and its final outcome. United States delegate Greg Jacob has argued that pressure from advocacy groups resulted in a treaty that has "remarkably little to do with international relations" and language "so broad as to be meaningless." "The framework model," he contended, "did not serve the needs of NGOs, the health ministers who were looking to force the hands of their governments, or trade lawyers who were looking for a little extra help in the trade courts." Instead, he claimed, "the groups in question undertook to pack the Convention full of all the substantive provisions that were on their wish list."[40]

From the outset of the treaty negotiations, the NGOs were intent on the idea of the FCTC serving as a floor, not a ceiling for international tobacco control standards. There was widespread recognition, however, that a weak, poorly defined treaty would be used by the tobacco industry to justify weak tobacco control measures at the national level. There was also concern that the international political attention given to tobacco at the time would not last and that there would be considerably less political pressure for countries to sign protocols in the future. It was imperative, the NGOs argued, that the draft text of the FCTC be as strong and specific as possible. Subsequent events have largely justified these concerns.

Contrary to Greg Jacob's assertions, NGOs did not achieve all of the provisions on their wish list. The language of the FCTC is generally framed as recommendations rather than the obligations that NGOs espoused. Inclusion of constitutional limitations weakened their efforts to impose a worldwide ban on advertising, promotion, and sponsorship of tobacco. NGOs failed in their efforts to ban descriptive terms on packaging such as *light* and *mild,* and to require pictograms in health warnings. The inability to secure language that prioritized health over trade was perhaps the NGOs' greatest failure, and it illustrates the tobacco industry's successful use of economic rationale to dissuade governments from enacting gold standard tobacco control policies domestically and at the international level.

Tobacco Industry Participation

WHO officially prohibited industry participation in the negotiations due to the substantial documentation showing that the industry had effectively blocked past WHO efforts to address the growing burden of tobacco-related disease.[41] Industry representatives complained about their limited involvement in the FCTC, claiming that WHO intended to ignore their companies and allies. Industry representatives were successful, however, in influencing the composition of national delegations, and, in some countries, obtaining a spot on the team.[42] Members of the industry are known to have been present on the national delegations of (at least) China, Japan, Malawi, Russia, and Turkey.

A key tactic employed by the industry to weaken national positions in relation to the FCTC was to influence the composition of national delegations. They pushed countries to include representatives from areas of the government where they had more influence, such as trade, finance, and agricultural ministries. Japan provides a particularly relevant example. At the first two INB sessions, Japan's delegation consisted mainly of representatives from the Ministry of Health, Welfare, and Labor, and it contained no representation from the Ministry of Finance. However, by INB6 there were as many representatives from the Ministry of Finance as there were representatives from the Ministry of Health, reflecting the importance of input from the tobacco industry.

The industry also hired private consultants and third-party organizations to engage in public relations. The most important of these organizations was the International Tobacco Growers' Association (ITGA). The ITGA received significant funding to promote the industry's point of view on the FCTC. The ITGA and consultants were especially useful in helping the industry frame the FCTC as economically harmful, a high-income country issue, and an affront to national sovereignty.

In addition to influencing national delegations and framing the debate, the industry also attempted to divert attention away from the FCTC through the development of youth smoking prevention and other voluntary programs. Sometime between 1999 and 2001, for example, BAT, Philip Morris, and JTI established Project Cerberus, a voluntary regulatory scheme for the tobacco industry that served as an alternative to the FCTC.[43] The aim of the project was to institute a voluntary regulatory code of practice that was overseen by an independent audit body, which focused primarily on preventing smoking among young people. Although the effort failed, the industry continued to promote its international tobacco product marketing standard and its youth prevention programs, despite evidence that they were ineffective at curbing tobacco use.

Industry activity was closely monitored by NGOs, who publicized the activity and pressured governments to reject industry influence. Members of NATT collected examples from around the world of industry efforts to affect countries' negotiating positions, and then used them in their lobbying and media advocacy efforts. The Zambia Consumer Association, for example, discovered that the tobacco industry had contacted the Zambian delegates by phone in Geneva to lobby for certain positions in their favor. The example was exposed in Infact's 2003 report, "Treaty Trespassers: New Evidence of Escalating Tobacco Industry Activity to Derail the Framework Convention on Tobacco Control," which sought to further dissuade governments from entering into dialogue with the tobacco industry.[44] In February 2003, protest letters were sent by members of the FCA and the NATT to President Bush after information leaked that the US embassy in Riyadh had sent a letter to the Saudi Arabian minister of foreign affairs arguing that the FCTC contradicted trade agreements and encouraging them to include the trade and agricultural ministries in developing their country's position during INB6.[45] The letter echoed the industry's strategy of involving these ministries in delegations to weaken the voice of health ministries.

Despite its supposed exclusion from the FCTC process, the presence of the tobacco industry was felt throughout the negotiations. Their arguments formed the backbone of many of the most contentious debates among countries, and their impact is obvious in the final text of many key provisions in the treaty.

Debate on Key Provisions in the Text

International treaty making has been described as "an art, not a science, and the results are usually finely-balanced, living documents that often have to respond to different constituencies in a number of jurisdictions with different concerns and policy priorities."[46] There is often a pronounced tendency toward lowest common denominator bargaining, where ambitious goals, mandated targets, and firm timelines are either removed or diluted. This was often the case in the FCTC negotiations and the fact that the negotiations were resolved by consensus and not by vote further required that countries accommodate weaker positions.

There were numerous key provisions in the draft treaty that created tension and resulted in bitter deliberations between those seeking binding commitments and those demanding optional text. In most cases, the lowest common denominator was victorious. Resistance from the United States and Germany to a complete ban on advertising, sponsorship, and promotion resulted in a comprehensive ban *or* restrictions in compliance with constitutional limitations. Japan and China's opposition to labeling and packaging requirements resulted in the replacement of a ban on terms such as *light* and *low tar* with labeling that does not promote a false, misleading, or erroneous impression and *may* include terms such as *light* or *mild*. The proposed requirement of pictograms in health warnings was also made voluntary. Strong opposition from Germany and Japan resulted in voluntary rather than mandatory prohibition of cigarette vending machines.

Although there were many issues throughout the negotiations that pitted countries against each other, perhaps none illustrates the divide better than the issue of trade and health. The industry's commitment to expanding markets in low- and middle-income countries made free and open trade crucial for the long-term health of tobacco companies. There was no other element of the FCTC that had the potential to undermine the growth of the transnational tobacco companies as much as trade did. The issue of trade also provided the industry with its best hope of derailing the entire FCTC; therefore, it pressed all levels of government to keep tobacco as a commodity under the World Trade Organization (WTO).

The World Bank report, while emphasizing the need to reduce demand for tobacco products rather than curtail their supply, concluded that trade liberalization has a large and significant impact on smoking in low-income countries, a smaller, but still important effect on smoking in middle-income countries, and no effect on high-income countries. The inequitable impact of trade liberalization highlighted by the report made the issue one of social equity and justice during the negotiations. Although the United States and Japan took the lead in fighting for industry-supported language prioritizing trade over health, the majority of other high-income countries also supported text that guaranteed the superiority of the WTO regime. Alternatively, a number of low- and middle-income countries argued for wording that prioritized health. Thailand was a key leader in this group. In the past it notoriously had been forced to open its market to transnational tobacco companies after it was challenged by the US trade representative in the General Agreement on Tariffs and Trade (GATT), the predecessor to the WTO. Throughout the FCTC negotiations, NGOs sided with Thailand and other low- and middle-income countries in arguing forcibly for specific language prioritizing public health over trade law.

Tension over the trade and health issue arose early in the negotiations. The working group's text included the language (later known as guiding principle D.5), "Trade policy measures for tobacco control purposes should not constitute a means of arbitrary or unjustifiable discrimination or a disguised restriction on international trade."[47] This proposal seemed to prioritize trade over health and was supported by major trading countries, including the United States, Germany, and Japan. It was also strongly supported by TFI because of TFI's primary objective to ensure successful negotiation of the FCTC. TFI maintained that "similar treaty language was contained in a number of multilateral environmental agreements" and that it was protective of public health.[48] In 2002, TFI released a report attempting to further clarify the issue, but the trade versus health debate continued to divide the public health community.

Responding to clear disagreement over guiding principle D.5, the "non-discrimination" trade provision, the chairman revised the text before INB4 to include four policy options. The options ranged from the FCTC taking precedence over all international agreements to subordination of the FCTC provision to previous international commitments. However, in October 2002 at INB5, guiding principle D.5 was replaced by articles 2.3 and 4.5, which further subordinated the FCTC to WTO.[49] Article 2.3 specifically stated, "Nothing in this Convention and its related protocols shall be interpreted as implying in any way a change in rights and obligations of a Party under any existing international treaty."[50] Article 4.5 stated, "While recognizing that tobacco control and trade measures can be implemented in a mutually supportive manner, Parties agree that tobacco control measures shall be transparent, implemented in accordance with their existing international obligations, and shall not constitute a means of arbitrary or unjustifiable discrimination in international trade."[51] This language resulted in intense backlash from NGOs and delegations that supported health over trade. TFI in particular was a target of the frustration because it was considered to be the source of the dramatic change in language. NGOs viewed TFI as bending to the United States and Japan and, consequently, the tobacco industry, rather than standing with the majority of member states who were pushing for public health.

According to individuals who were part of TFI at the time, it was Brundtland who instructed TFI leadership during a closed meeting to do what was needed to assure that trade was not included in the final treaty. Reportedly a number of high-income country supporters of the treaty had made it clear to her that trade language would be a major impediment to their ability to adopt the treaty. She was also allegedly concerned that trade language would rattle the pharmaceutical industry, which was engaged at the time in heated battles over patent rights and drug access for HIV patients in low- and middle-income countries. There was an overall feeling among individuals in the secretariat that NGOs did not understand that countries, including Germany, the United States, the United Kingdom, Australia, China, and other members of the European Union, would have walked away from the negotiations if health was prioritized over trade in the treaty.

The dispute over trade-related language in the text provided a key moment for the development of the Framework Convention Alliance. Given the origins of the FCA, TFI had historically seen itself as a parent figure to the group. Although it kept the FCA at arms' length, TFI clearly understood the value of having a strong and influential civil society presence supporting the FCTC, especially when it came to supporting TFI's capacity-building and educational activities. However, the FCA was now an aggressive challenger that was not afraid to pick a political fight with the secretariat. The FCA hired its own trade consultants and directly challenged TFI's expertise on the issue. Members of TFI were shocked and infuriated by the FCA's challenge, and the relationship between the two organizations soured. Although relations subsequently have improved between the two, the FCA's independence was clearly established at this time and it has since been respected as a powerful political force.

Between INB5 and INB6, the contentious articles 2.3 and 4.5 that subordinated the FCTC to WTO were deleted based on the argument that previous international conventions already dealt with relationships between treaties. The Vienna Convention on the Law of Treaties, for example, stipulated that "the more recent treaty will be applied in precedence over the older one" and "the more specific treaty will be applied in precedence over the more general one."[52] In an unpublished briefing note to the chair, TFI suggested that because the FCTC was more recent and product specific, it would supersede older and more generic treaties, including WTO. NGOs vigorously disagreed and convinced the chair to reinsert both articles in the INB6 text to allow for revision favoring specific health over trade language. Latin American countries, who were initially supportive of guiding principle D.5, grew increasingly supportive of health over trade language as the negotiations progressed, and they became a key ally to Thailand during INB6.[53]

In the end, consensus between the two blocks could not be reached, and the "silence" proposal from TFI gained reluctant support from both sides. In the *Alliance Bulletin* during INB6, FCA trade consultant Ira Shapiro wrote that the FCA has "steadfastly supported a clear statement that the public health provision of the FCTC should prevail over the general trade rules of WTO when and if conflicts arise. . . . But if delegates can't get it right, then it's better to say nothing at all."[54] However, even as the FCA came to recognize that it was not going to get an explicit clause allowing health to trump trade, it still criticized the general beliefs among delegates that there probably would not be conflicts between the FCTC and trade agreements, and that if there were, the trade–health conflicts would be resolved in favor of health.

The belief among delegates that health would be recognized as a priority by WTO was based on the first line of the FCTC's preamble, "The Parties to this Convention, Determined to give priority to their right to protect public health." This language was reflective of a similar approach taken by the Codex Alimentarius Commission (jointly led by WHO and the Food and Agricultural Organization) for food safety, labeling, and advertising aimed at informing future trade disputes. WHO officials worked behind the scenes to obtain unofficial support from WTO for this interpretation of the treaty. Following the end of negotiations on March 7, 2003, Supachai Panitchpakdi, then director general of WTO, released a statement in which he stated: "I congratulate all of those who worked so hard to bring about this important agreement. . . . When dealing with the pressing problems of our age, whether they are related to improving health standards or eradicating poverty, there can be no doubt that the nations of the world must work together."[55] This announcement, WHO argued, was evidence that the highest levels of the global trade regime had heard and acknowledged the public health goals behind the FCTC.[56]

Unfortunately, the stance of the FCA has proven more accurate over time as trade disputes have become a defining feature of tobacco control efforts in the post-FCTC world. The FCTC's failure to specifically address public health versus trade liberalization has provided the space for the tobacco industry to challenge national tobacco control policies under investment and trade treaties. Even if decisions are eventually reached that support national tobacco control policies that are applied in a non-discriminatory manner, the confusion and uncertainty surrounding ongoing litigation has undercut national efforts, stalled global momentum, and delayed aggressive action in many countries.

The failure to address trade also suggests that the FCTC failed to address the major transnational driver of the tobacco epidemic, and thus partially failed its original objective to improve transnational tobacco control policy coherence. The FCTC's silence on trade also highlights the difficulties of ensuring policy coherence across global health, development, and economic policies within and between countries.[57] Above all, the failure to find consensus around trade reflects the overwhelming primacy afforded to trade liberalization by the United States and other high-income countries and the continued viability of the transnational tobacco industry. Although highly unlikely, there is still a possibility that WHO could develop a protocol to deal with the broader trade–health issue in the long term. The rise in trade disputes certainly points to the growing need for further clarity in the matter. A deeper discussion of recent trade litigation and the impact of decisions reached on the ability of countries to adopt strong, effective, and comprehensive tobacco control policies is provided in subsequent chapters.

Adoption of the Final Treaty Text

As the FCTC negotiations came to an end, there remained one last unresolved issue. The United States and Germany argued forcibly that a reservations clause should be included in the treaty. Such a clause would allow countries to ratify the convention but elect to be bound only by specific provisions of their choosing. However, after having compromised on nearly every other key provision, the vast majority of member states countered that allowing such reservations would make the treaty essentially meaningless. To further isolate the United States' position, NGOs capitalized on the international unpopularity of the US military intervention in Iraq. These broader political events at the time emboldened member states that would otherwise not have stood up against the United States and supported the treaty. It was clear that the block of low- and middle-income countries, strongly supported by civil society, would not back down from their insistence on the exclusion of a reservations clause. The final decision to not allow reservations distinguishes the FCTC from most other global treaties and was a key victory over those seeking to undermine the impact of the (increasingly weakened) FCTC text.

Following the end of negotiations in February 2003, there remained strong opposition to the treaty from the United States and Germany. Both argued that the inclusion of a comprehensive advertising ban was unacceptable despite language acknowledging that some country constitutions limited the potential scope of such bans. They also continued to insist on a reservations clause that allowed countries to pick and choose acceptable items from the treaty. The ball was now in their court: they could either go along with the global majority or oppose the global agreement in front of the world at the upcoming fifty-sixth WHA.

On the eve of the World Health Assembly in May, with indications of a show-down between the United States and the rest of the world, then US Secretary of Health and Human Services Tommy Thompson held a news conference to announce that the United States would accept the final text as written. Shortly thereafter the German minister of health also expressed Germany's willingness to accept the treaty.

The reasons for the last-minute turnaround of the United States and Germany on the FCTC final text are not clear. Some have speculated that the United States did not want to endure additional international criticism for obstructing global public health while it was already engaged in an unpopular war. Others hypothesize that the tobacco industry in these countries eventually concluded that the treaty did not represent a sufficient threat to warrant the political fight against it. When asked by reporters for an explanation for the surprise shift in the US position, Thompson gave only a short, cryptic response: "Someday I will tell you."[58] Whether the deciding factor was intense NGO lobbying or a "go ahead" signal from the tobacco industry is unknown.

On May 21, 2003, the fifty-sixth WHA unanimously adopted the WHO Framework Convention on Tobacco Control.[59] Many universal elements of national tobacco control policy are included as core provisions in the final text, representing a victory for those advocating for a strong, comprehensive treaty. The preamble of the WHO FCTC gives due regard to the right to protect public health, the global nature of the tobacco epidemic, the increase in global consumption of tobacco products, the scientific evidence of the harm caused by tobacco use and exposure to tobacco smoke, and the social, economic, and environmental consequences of tobacco consumption.

Parties to the WHO FCTC also recognized the "need to be alert to any efforts by the tobacco industry to undermine or subvert tobacco control efforts and the need to be informed of activities of the tobacco industry that have a negative impact on tobacco efforts."[60] The objective of the WHO FCTC, outlined in article 3, is "to protect present and future generations from the devastating health, social, environmental and economic consequences of tobacco consumption and exposure to tobacco smoke by providing a framework for tobacco control measures . . . in order to reduce continually and substantially the prevalence of tobacco use and exposure to tobacco smoke."[61]

The WHO FCTC emphasizes demand reduction strategies. The core demand reduction provisions are contained in articles 6 to 14, whereas supply reduction provisions are set out in articles 15 to 17.[62] Novel features of the treaty include the provisions that address liability of the tobacco industry (article 19), mechanisms

TABLE 2
Key Demand Reduction Provisions of the FCTC

Article	Description
6: Price and tax measures to reduce the demand for tobacco	Recognizes that price and tax measures are an effective and important means of reducing tobacco consumption, especially among young people.
8: Protection from exposure to tobacco smoke	Requires parties to adopt and implement effective measures providing for protection from exposure to tobacco smoke in indoor workplaces, public transport, indoor public places, and, as appropriate, other public places.
9: Regulation of the contents of tobacco products	Obligates countries to require manufacturers and importers of tobacco products to disclose to governmental authorities information about product contents and emissions. Measures for public disclosure must be adopted.
10: Regulation of tobacco product disclosures	Conference of the parties is to develop guidelines that can be used by countries for testing, measuring, and regulating contents and emissions. Parties must adopt pertinent measures at the national level.
11: Packaging and labeling of tobacco products	Requires parties to adopt and implement effective measures requiring large, clear health warnings, and to use rotating messages approved by a designated national authority. Provides that these warnings should cover 50% or more of the principal display areas and must occupy at least 30%. Also requires parties to adopt and implement effective measures to ensure that tobacco product packaging and labeling does not promote a tobacco product by any means that are false, misleading, deceptive, or likely to create an erroneous impression about its characteristics, health effects, hazards, or emissions.
12: Education, communication, training, and public awareness	Requires the adoption of legislative, executive, administrative, or other measures that promote public awareness and access to information on the addictiveness of tobacco, the health risks of tobacco use and exposure to smoke, the benefits of cessation, and the actions of the tobacco industry.
13: Tobacco advertising, promotion, and sponsorship	Requires, in accordance with constitutional limitations, a comprehensive ban on all tobacco advertising, promotion, and sponsorship.
14: Demand reduction measures concerning tobacco dependence and cessation	Requires creation of cessation programs in a range of settings. Includes diagnosis and treatment of nicotine dependence in national health programs, establishment of programs for diagnosis, and counseling and treatment in healthcare facilities and rehabilitation centers.

for scientific and technical cooperation and exchange of information (articles 20 to 22), and the importance of civil society participation as "essential in achieving the objective of the Convention and its protocols" (article 4.7).[63]

Key provisions include a *comprehensive* (as opposed to complete) ban on tobacco advertising, promotion, and sponsorship (with an exception for countries with constitutional limitations) (article 13); a ban on misleading descriptors that convince smokers that certain products are safer than standard cigarettes (which may include the terms *mild* and *light*) (article 11); and a mandate to place rotating warnings that cover at least 30% of tobacco packaging, with encouragement for even larger, graphic warnings (article 11). The WHO FCTC also mandates countries to implement smoke-free public place laws (article 8) and encourages them to address tobacco smuggling (article 15) and to increase tobacco taxes (article 6).

Remarkably, the FCTC is weakest when it comes to cross-border aspects of tobacco control. There are no binding obligations in relation to price, no agreement on synchronization of price levels, and no binding commitments regarding transnational advertising. Duty-free cigarettes remained legal, and the word *trade* never appears in the FCTC. In regard to price harmonization, there was very little debate; nearly all countries agreed that it was a sovereign right of states to determine their own fiscal policy. As such, the FCTC is much less a tool of international law than an agreement between states to institute domestic law based on common values related to the control and prevention of tobacco-related disease. At INB5, the WHO director general acknowledged that the text of the treaty was falling far short of her initial expectations; however, by INB6 Brundtland was appealing for countries to support a draft that could command broad support. At this they were successful.

Signature and Ratification

The FCTC was opened for signature on June 16, 2003, and closed on June 22, 2003, with 168 signatories, making it one of the most widely embraced global treaties in history. Signing the treaty was a political act that indicated a member state's intent to ratify it and to not oppose implementation of provisions of the treaty by other states. Signature was not the same as ratification, which made the treaty binding within a country. Each of the Big Four (Japan, Germany, United States, and China) signed the treaty. Notable non-signatories included Russia, which acceded to the treaty in 2008 after intense domestic and international lobbying, and Indonesia, which remains a non-party to the treaty.

In addition to signature, at least 40 member states had to ratify, accept, approve, formally consent, and accede to the treaty for the FCTC to enter into force. Ratification, acceptance, approval, and accession are all terms signifying an act by which a state, depending on country procedures, expresses its consent to be bound by a treaty. Accession differs from the other three actions in that it is a method used by a state that wishes to become a party to a treaty but did not sign before the period for signature elapsed. On November 29, 2004, the fortieth instrument of ratification, acceptance, approval, formal confirmation, or accession was deposited at UN headquarters. Ninety days later, on February 27, 2005, the WHO FCTC entered into force. This short time period makes the WHO FCTC among the fastest treaties in history to be negotiated, adopted, and entered into force.[64]

Ratification rapidly continued over the following years with active technical support from WHO and the FCA (see Appendix: Ratification of the FCTC). Ten years after its adoption by the WHA, 176 countries had ratified the treaty, representing 88.6% of the world's population. Only two highly populous countries in the world had not become party to the convention: the United States and Indonesia. Another notable non-party was Switzerland, the relatively new home to the headquarters of Philip Morris International and Japan Tobacco International. The extraordinary number of ratifications of the treaty in all regions of the world is seen by many and described by former INB Chair Amorim as "self-evidence that the whole [FCTC] exercise was highly successful."[65]

However, ratification has not always been seen as an indication of the treaty's value. Japan, for example, was among the first 40 countries to ratify the treaty. At no point within the negotiations did Japan budge in its opposition to key provisions in the FCTC text, including the total ban on advertising, prohibition of the use of descriptors such as *light* and *mild* cigarettes, and any provision in the FCTC that would allow public health to take precedence over trade.[66] Japan's last-minute decision to adopt the FCTC in May 2003 was understood by most as an attempt not to be seen as one of the few countries opposed to the FCTC. Its surprisingly rapid decision to be a party to the FCTC was not seen as a sudden awakening to the benefits of tobacco control, but as assurance of its ability to influence the treaty's implementation. Likewise, China and Germany ratified the treaty in 2004, although the grounds for their participation were mixed, and implementation in both countries has been challenging as described in Part II of this book. The willingness of Japan, China, and Germany to ratify the treaty likely reflects the optional, rather than obligatory, language in the text and their desire to have a vote in its implementation.

CHAPTER FOUR

With Force

The First Decade of FCTC Implementation

The entry into force of the Framework Convention on Tobacco Control in February 2005 marked a new phase for global tobacco control. Once considered a long shot, success of the treaty now rested in ensuring that the obligations and commitments made under the treaty were successfully translated into effective international institutions and national legislation and programs. The negotiation process had resulted in increased awareness about tobacco control and had generated political buy-in within countries. It had also consolidated a strong and effective global civil society movement in support of the treaty. However, new challenges quickly arose that threatened the treaty's progress, including financial downturns, competing political and fiscal priorities, and a rebound of the tobacco industry's image. New tactics and new financial resources would become key in the treaty's first decade.

Global FCTC Implementation

Resolution WHA56.1, the same resolution in which the FCTC was adopted, set out the initial steps for implementing the treaty, including the establishment of an open-ended intergovernmental working group.[1] The resolution also maintained that the interim secretariat for the working group should remain within the World Health Organization, and member states requested that Ambassador Luiz Felipe de Seixas Corrêa continue to serve as chair. The working group held two sessions in 2004 and 2005 in which it outlined the procedures necessary for implementation of the treaty. Following the FCTC's fortieth ratification and entry into force, the working group was replaced by the Conference of Parties (COP).

Conference of Parties

The COP is the main decision-making body established by the FCTC that is responsible for reviewing global implementation of the convention and driving

TABLE 3
Timeline of Meetings by the COP and the INB

Meeting	Date	Location	No. of Countries Participating
COP1	February 6–17, 2006	Geneva, Switzerland	109
COP2	June 30–July 6, 2007	Bangkok, Thailand	129
INB1	February 11–16, 2008	Geneva, Switzerland	132
INB2	October 20–25, 2008	Geneva, Switzerland	133
COP3	November 17–22, 2008	Durban, South Africa	130
INB3	June 28–July 5, 2009	Geneva, Switzerland	136
INB4	March 14–21, 2010	Geneva, Switzerland	141
COP4	November 15–20, 2010	Punta del Este, Uruguay	137
INB5	March 29–April 4, 2012	Geneva, Switzerland	133
COP5	November 12–17, 2012	Seoul, South Korea	136

COP indicates Conference of Parties to the WHO Framework Convention on Tobacco Control; INB, Intergovernmental Negotiating Body on a Protocol on Illicit Trade in Tobacco Products.
Data from the Framework Convention Alliance.

forward effective implementation of its provisions. The COP held its first session in Geneva on February 6–17, 2006, at which time 116 countries had ratified the FCTC, including many of the treaty's strongest critics, such as Japan, China, and Germany. The first COP made a number of key decisions regarding the implementation of the treaty. It was decided, for example, that the permanent secretariat of the convention should be established by WHO in Geneva. On June 1, 2007, the WHO director general announced the appointment of Haik Nikogosian as the head of the convention secretariat for an initial four-year term.[2] Nikogosian was subsequently reappointed for a second term, thus leading the convention secretariat for its first eight years. Subsequent COPs were held in Bangkok, Thailand (2007), Durban, South Africa (2008), Punta del Este, Uruguay (2010), and Seoul, South Korea (2012).[3] The COP made many important decisions at each of these sessions, particularly in regard to implementation guidelines and reporting.

KEY COP DECISIONS: GUIDELINES AND REPORTING

Development and approval of implementation guidelines comprised a core element of the COP's initial workload. Based on FCTC article 7, COP1 initiated work on guidelines for the implementation of the convention. Guidelines are not legally binding, but by unanimously adopting guidelines, all parties agree to the principles, definitions, and factual findings contained within them. Coupled with the legal duty to interpret the treaty in good faith, this means that FCTC member countries should view the adopted guidelines as a practical description of what is necessary to meet their obligations under the FCTC and the standards against which parties' implementation should be judged. The COP has established a

TABLE 4
COP Guidelines

Article	Issue	Date of Adoption	Meeting
5.3	The protection of public health policies with respect to tobacco control from commercial and other vested interests	November 2008	COP3
8	The protection from exposure to tobacco smoke	July 2007	COP2
9, 10	Regulation of the contents of tobacco products and regulation of tobacco product disclosures (partial guidelines)	November 2010 and 2012	COP4/COP5
11	Packaging and labeling of tobacco products	November 2008	COP3
12	Education, communication, training, and public awareness	November 2010	COP4
13	Tobacco advertising, promotion, and sponsorship	November 2008	COP3
14	Demand reduction measures concerning tobacco dependence and cessation	November 2010	COP4

Data from the World Health Organization.

number of intersessional working groups to develop guidelines and recommendations for the implementation of different treaty provisions. The working groups involve a wide consultative and intergovernmental process, which is determined at the discretion of each group.

Guidelines covering a wide range of provisions within the treaty (addressing seven articles in total) were adopted by the COP at its second through fifth sessions. Discussions about potential future guidelines in advance of COP6 focused on economically sustainable alternatives to tobacco growing (articles 17 and 18) and price and tax measures to reduce the demand for tobacco (article 6). The guidelines are a critical tool for tobacco control advocates in their work to ensure that governments meet their obligations and act as effectively as possible to protect the public from the devastating effects of the tobacco epidemic.

Beginning at COP1, a number of decisions were made in regard to obligations under article 21 of the convention concerning when and how countries should report their progress in implementing the FCTC. The objective of reporting is to enable parties to learn from each other's experiences in implementing the treaty, and the reports serve as the basis by which the COP reviews progress in implementing the convention worldwide.[4] From 2007 to 2011, party reports were submitted according to the first (group 1 questions) and second (group 2 questions) phases of the reporting instrument adopted by the COP at its first and third sessions, respectively.

There was debate within the COP that reporting was overly burdensome on countries and, in November 2010 at its fourth session, the COP decided to adopt a single reporting instrument for parties' biennial reports.[5] The reporting instrument consists of a core questionnaire that is mandatory for all parties and the "additional questions on the use of implementation guidelines adopted by the Conference of the Parties," which aim to facilitate voluntary submission of such information by the parties.[6] Parties also decided at COP4 that implementation reports should be submitted at regular two-year intervals, synchronized with the cycle of the regular sessions of the COP.

By 2014, more than 80% of parties had submitted at least one report to the secretariat, with many having multiple reports on file.[7] All implementation reports and the annexes to those reports are available to the public on the convention secretariat website.[8] The convention secretariat also maintains a WHO FCTC implementation database containing all data reported by parties.[9] The database is searchable by party, by specific treaty articles, or by individual measures. The reports have been heavily criticized, however, by representatives of civil society for being overly positive and lacking validation. The COP continues to focus on improving the process and debating if and how non-state actors may contribute to the reporting process.

COP PARTICIPATION

Participation in the COP has been extremely strong, with hundreds of state and non-state participants at each session. Ninety-five percent of parties to the FCTC participated in at least one of the first four sessions of the COP, with the proportion of parties attending each session typically more than 80% across most income groups and regions.[10] An additional 23 countries who had not yet ratified the treaty attended at least one of the first five COPs as observers (without a right to vote). There was, however, a decline in attendance at COP meetings over time. The proportion of participating parties dropped from 95% in 2006 to 80% in 2010. This decline was most pronounced among higher middle-income countries and may reflect a decline in the political priority afforded tobacco control in the context of the global financial crisis of the time.[11]

Low- and middle-income countries have not only been present at the COP sessions, but have had significant influence on its decisions. A key aspect of the COP negotiations is the "one party, one vote" rule. That is, any country, big or small, has the same right to be heard, and the same number of votes, so long as it has ratified the treaty and is a party. Consequently, even tiny countries can and have wielded influence far beyond their size or gross domestic product.[12] Alternatively, the United States joins Argentina, Indonesia, and a number of other non-ratifying countries as observers in the very back of the room.

The experience that small and lower-income countries gained standing up to powerful countries' interests during the FCTC negotiations increased their ability to influence COP outcomes. Canadian tobacco control advocate and FCA Director of Policy and Advocacy, Frances Thompson, has described how smaller, lower-income countries have successfully forced the European Union, Japan, and China to make considerable concessions in the development of guidelines.[13] For example, going into the third COP in Durban, the draft 5.3 guidelines on preventing tobacco industry interference included language supported by the tobacco-friendly states and the European Union: "governments should interact with the tobacco industry only when necessary, in line with the principle of good governance."[14] Delegates of many lower-income countries feared that this line could be interpreted as meaning that the tobacco industry should be consulted on virtually anything that affects their interest. Led by Oman (population three million), these countries forcefully defended their interests and were successful in sending stronger guidelines back to the plenary for adoption.[15]

Participation of low- and middle-income countries has been strong in part due to a travel policy providing an economy air ticket and per diem expenses for one delegate from these countries to all COP meetings. Moreover, the rotating location of the COP sessions across the WHO regions has facilitated access to the meetings. Decisions at COP5 to consider rolling back this funding support and to host future sessions in Europe (a request championed by the European region) may have a lasting impact on the COP, reducing the participation of smaller, lower-income countries and challenging the social justice record of the convention.[16]

As was the case during the FCTC negotiations, civil society has actively participated in the COP. At the 115th session of the WHO executive board in February 2005, the FCA entered into formal relations with WHO.[17] The FCA has since had an official presence at all COP sessions, which has helped it better control its own policy platforms and has increased the number of delegates permitted to attend the sessions. In many cases, the FCA has taken an active role in the development of the implementation guidelines, although its precise access to, and role in, the process differs according to the decisions of each group. At each COP session, the FCA has continued to carry out its advocacy and technical assistance activities, including revealing the "death clock" (also a constant fixture on its website) and producing the daily *Alliance Bulletin* (as it did for all sessions of the Intergovernmental Negotiating Body on a Protocol on Illicit Trade in Tobacco

Products, described later in this chapter). The Orchid and Dirty Ashtray Awards remained influential symbols in the COP process, and the FCA continued to engage regionally and within countries to prepare for global negotiations, even providing financial support for government delegates from NGO-friendly, low-income countries.

With philanthropic support, the FCA established a global tobacco control policy monitoring system that tracks the status and progress of implementation of effective tobacco control measures. *Tobacco Watch*, produced in advance of the COP sessions, builds on the information provided by the countries in their official reports to the secretariat and includes observational data based on the input of tobacco control advocates in those countries.[18] The FCA has used *Tobacco Watch* to call for stronger enforcement of and compliance with FCTC-related policies, and points to its findings as evidence for the need to strengthen the official reporting process.

NON-PARTIES

At the end of 2013, 177 WHO member states were party to the treaty, comprising 88% of the world's population.[19] Significant non-parties remained, including the United States, Indonesia, and Argentina. Given the population size and prevalence of tobacco use in these countries, their absence from the treaty directly challenged the FCTC's global impact. There is some disagreement, however, over whether their accession to the treaty and formal participation in the COP would be good for the treaty, or if it would obstruct efforts to effectively implement the treaty provisions. This argument has particular relevance in regard to the United States.

Throughout the FCTC negotiations, many US-based members of civil society argued that concessions should not be made to the United States because it was highly unlikely that the United States would ever become party to the treaty.[20] This belief was based on the United States' poor record in joining international legal agreements. Other noteworthy international treaties that the United States is not party to include the Convention to Eliminate All Forms of Discrimination Against Women, the Convention on the Rights of the Child, the International Covenant on Economic, Social and Cultural Rights, the Comprehensive Test Ban Treaty, and the Mine Ban Treaty.

As anticipated, the US Senate did not ratify the FCTC, although it did not reject it. As of 2014, the FCTC remains "in review" by the State Department, having never been forwarded to the Senate by the White House. President Obama expressed a strong commitment to the FCTC as a member of the US Senate when he joined a letter to then President Bush urging him to send the treaty to the Senate for consideration.[21] The letter stated, "the FCTC is a historic opportunity to protect current and future generations both at home and abroad from some of the devastating consequences of tobacco use. The United States must be up to the challenge of turning this opportunity into a reality."[22] Since entering presidential office, however, Obama has failed to send the treaty to Congress. There was some speculation that he would move on the treaty if, and when, the Family Smoking and Prevention Act was approved by Congress. This act officially gives the US Food and Drug Administration authority over tobacco and brings US law in line with all binding obligations within the treaty. It passed and entered into force in 2009,[23] but Obama has still failed to submit the treaty for a Senate vote.

There are multiple hypotheses for why Obama has not sent the FCTC to the Senate. The primary hypothesis is that he and his advisors believe that the Senate, as currently composed, cannot muster the two-thirds majority needed to approve the treaty. It would be highly embarrassing for Obama (and most Americans) to have the United States officially on record as voting against the world's first, and widely accepted, public health treaty. Silence on the matter seems to be preferable.

Generally speaking, there has been little civil society pressure on the United States to ratify the treaty, likely reflecting the overriding belief that the treaty has little chance of approval in the US Senate. Fears also persist that US participation would serve as a stumbling block in the COP as it was during the FCTC negotiations. The same cannot be said for Argentina and Indonesia, where international and domestic activists have been working for years, and in Indonesia investing millions of dollars, to push the FCTC forward. The tobacco industry wields considerable influence in both countries. Indonesia has a large tobacco industry and has long resisted domestic tobacco control efforts. Between 2009 and 2012, tobacco consumption in Indonesia increased annually, making it home to the third highest number of smokers in the world after China and India.[24] However, the press continues to report on progress toward ratification. In 2013, the Indonesia Tobacco Control Network launched a "roadmap" to accelerate ratification.[25] President Susilo Bambang Yudhoyono reportedly agreed in principle to ratification but wanted the government to speak with one voice on the subject.[26]

In 2011, Argentina passed a National Tobacco Control Law but did not develop the required regulations to properly implement the law, and the FCTC was not ratified.[27] Research has shown that tobacco producers and transnational tobacco companies successfully built opposition to FCTC ratification in Argentina by lobbying provincial legislators and federal officials from the Ministry of the Economy and by placing stories in regional media to obstruct approval of tobacco control laws.[28] According to an Argentinian tobacco growing association, the FCTC was mentioned in regional newspapers three to seven times per week in 2009 in articles about alleged adverse economic effects of tobacco control.[29] International efforts were made to counteract these arguments. In 2009, Haik Nikogosian, head of the FCTC secretariat, visited Argentina to mobilize civil society and lawmakers sitting on the legislative health committees.[30] The FCA repeatedly called on Argentina to ratify the treaty, arguing that it is isolating itself and losing the opportunity to participate in the development of the treaty. Advocates also took advantage of the location of COP4 in neighbouring Uruguay to highlight Argentina's position as the only non-party in South America. Such efforts have thus far been unsuccessful.

Intergovernmental Negotiating Body on a Protocol on Illicit Trade in Tobacco Products

Reflecting on the COP process, Paula Jones, a tobacco control activist from Brazil, has noted a significant shift in the attitude and approach to the negotiations among delegates at the COPs relative to the INBs.[31] The overriding feelings of "this is impossible" or "we have no idea where we are heading" experienced at the beginning of the FCTC negotiations, Jones argues, were replaced by feelings of "yes, we can do it" and "many countries are doing it."[32] This enthusiasm, however, has not been reflected in the COP's decisions to move forward on the development of strong, binding protocols to the FCTC. At the end of the sixth INB, parties agreed to postpone the discussion on protocols until after the treaty was adopted. Despite proposals for multiple protocols at the first COP, nearly a decade after the FCTC's entry into force, only one protocol had been negotiated and adopted. It appears that advocates were correct in their early fears that the FCTC negotiations presented a unique window of opportunity to mobilize binding commitments from member states.

To date, the COP has only used its right, in accordance with article 33 of the convention, to adopt one protocol to the FCTC: a protocol on illicit trade in tobacco products. The decision to move forward on the protocol was first made at the second COP in Bangkok in 2007.[33] The COP subsequently established an Intergovernmental Negotiating Body on a Protocol on Illicit Trade in Tobacco Products. Negotiations began in 2008 and, after five negotiating sessions, the final text of the Protocol to Eliminate Illicit Trade in Tobacco Products was adopted at COP5 in November 2012.[34]

The objective of the protocol is to eliminate all forms of illicit trade in tobacco products by requiring parties to take measures to effectively control the supply chain of tobacco products and to cooperate internationally on a wide range of matters.[35] Part III of the protocol, "Supply Chain Control," contains provisions on licensing, due diligence, tracking and tracing, record-keeping, security and preventive measures, sale by internet, telecommunication, or any other evolving technology, free zones and international transit, and duty-free sales. During the negotiations, Part III was referred to as the "heart" of the protocol.[36] Other important provisions cover offences, seizure payments, and disposal/destruction of confiscated products.

In accordance with its article 43, the protocol was open for signature by all parties to the WHO FCTC from January 10, 2013, to January 9, 2014. When it was closed for signature, the protocol had been signed by 53 states and the European Union.[37] Like the FCTC, the illicit trade protocol will enter into force on the ninetieth day after the date of deposit of the fortieth instrument of ratification, acceptance, approval, formal confirmation, or accession with the depositary (article 45). This date does not appear to be quickly approaching: one year after its adoption, only one country (Nicaragua) had ratified the protocol.

There are many arguments for why the protocol was not quickly ratified. Some point to the convention secretariat, who took very little action to follow up on the adoption of the protocol and push parties to ratify. However, there are a number of technical reasons for the reluctance of parties to ratify the protocol. The protocol is, based on its content, essentially a customs and law enforcement treaty created by a health institution.[38] The protocol's preamble recognizes the need to enhance cooperation among the protocol's secretariat, which is also the convention secretariat, the UN Office on Drugs and Crime, the World Customs Organization (WCO), and other bodies. The protocol calls for the cooperation of competent international and regional intergovernmental organizations in its governing body, the Meeting of the Parties (MOP), to provide technical and financial support to achieve its objective. Yet it is not clear how the convention secretariat or the tobacco units in WHO and regional offices will be able to facilitate the protocol's implementation.[39]

Anticipating the protocol's adoption, the convention secretariat developed a document outlining the activities and budget required for preparation of its entry into force for the COP's consideration. The secretariat, the document stated, would "utiliz[e] existing capacity" but would "require some additional capacity to carry out the protocol-related tasks."[40] Additional staff would be required to cover protocol-specific issues that are not currently covered by the secretariat, including matters related to customs and supply chain control, criminal law and law enforcement, and technology issues related to global information sharing. In other words, the secretariat did not have the expertise in house to implement the heart of the protocol. The document proposed the addition of three professional staff, "one per area of expertise," and two administrative staff, to carry out the work. The COP, however, secured less than the cost of employing one qualified staff member for one year.

In the absence of financial and human resources for the secretariat, the European Union, the protocol's primary originator and financial supporter, distributed a "roadmap for carrying out priority tasks for the implementation of the protocol," which called for the assessment of each article of the protocol to determine how to implement its provisions.[41] This assessment was to be farmed out to party experts who had been involved in the protocol discussions—once again reflecting the lack of subject matter expertise by the convention secretariat in the core areas of the protocol.

Another important sticking point for many parties in relation to the protocol was the potential involvement of the tobacco industry in its implementation. Both Philip Morris International (PMI) and British American Tobacco (BAT) welcomed the protocol's adoption. The industry's approval was met with intense suspicion from civil society and many parties. It is widely acknowledged that the tobacco industry sees illicit trade as an area in which it can portray itself as a partner of governments and intergovernmental organizations and legitimize itself as an ordinary private sector entity. In sharp contrast to WHO, the international agencies that have the expertise and capacity to facilitate and support activity to combat illicit trade, such as the World Customs Organization and the International Criminal Police Organization (INTERPOL), view the tobacco industry as a legitimate private industry stakeholder with whom they cooperate closely. INTERPOL, for example, applied for intergovernmental organization observer status with the COP, stating that it believed that it could "play an important role in assisting the parties to the WHO FCTC, the majority of which are also member countries of INTERPOL, to coordinate and facilitate international cooperation to eliminate illicit trade in tobacco products."[42] During COP4, however, parties decided to defer INTERPOL's application after controversy arose over INTERPOL's relationship with the tobacco industry. Just prior to COP4, INTERPOL's general counsel and legal officer published an article arguing that:

> Any success against the ITTP [illicit trade in tobacco products] requires that law enforcement and national authorities work together with the legitimate tobacco industry for a number of reasons. Tobacco companies are able to assist

governments in different aspects, including providing resources to enhance capacity, providing technical assistance such as schemes to distinguish genuine tobacco products from counterfeit products and training customs officials in relation to contraband products.[43]

Moreover, on June 12, 2012, INTERPOL accepted a pledge of €15 million over three years from PMI.

Given these concerns, parties have argued that implementation of the protocol threatens to overtake other parts of the FCTC in terms of attention, budget, and personnel; dilutes the norms and values of the treaty; and should be tabled. Consequently, the protocol is still far from becoming a binding international treaty and represents a less than successful chapter in the FCTC's development.

Bloomberg Initiative to Reduce Tobacco Use and MPOWER

In late 2006, New York City Mayor Michael Bloomberg announced his intention to fund a major global tobacco control initiative.[44] Bloomberg had become well known for his support for public health in general, including his endowment of the Johns Hopkins School of Public Health, now known as the Johns Hopkins Bloomberg School of Public Health, and for his support for tobacco control in particular. As mayor of New York City, he oversaw the passage and enforcement of the city's complete smoking ban, which he has claimed to be his greatest achievement in office. During his tenure, Bloomberg succeeded in raising tobacco taxes, launching hard-hitting public education campaigns, creating tobacco cessation support programs, and rigorously monitoring smoking rates. The city's tobacco control program was effective, reducing adult smoking prevalence from 21.6% in 2002 to 16.9% in 2007.[45] Teen smoking decreased from 17.6% in 2001 to 8.5% in 2007, a level nearly two-thirds lower than the US national average at the time.[46]

Building on this legacy in tobacco control, Bloomberg decided to invest a significant portion of his personal wealth in the global fight to prevent and control tobacco use. The Bloomberg Initiative to Reduce Tobacco Use was formally launched in early 2007 with an initial commitment of $125 million. The initiative was first led by Tom Frieden, then New York City health commissioner (and future director of the Centers for Disease Control and Prevention), and was administered through five partner institutions: the Campaign for Tobacco-Free Kids, the CDC Foundation, the Johns Hopkins Bloomberg School of Public Health, the World Lung Foundation, and WHO.[47]

In 2008, Bill Gates strayed from his adherence to global health issues related to vaccines and maternal and child health to join Bloomberg in funding the initiative's work, bringing the initiative's overall funding to more than $500 million.[48] In 2012, Bloomberg increased his personal investment in the initiative again, committing an additional $220 million over four years and bringing his personal commitment to more than $600 million.[49]

From the beginning, the initiative was primarily targeted at large, heavily populated low- and middle-income countries with high smoking rates, in particular China, India, Indonesia, Russia, and Bangladesh. A key aspect of the initiative was its competitive grants program, which awarded more than 125 grants in 36 countries in its first five years.[50] The Bloomberg Initiative also targeted training programs, journalism workshops, in-country development of mass media public education campaigns, and capacity building. The Global Tobacco Control Leadership Program, a two-week summer course held at the Bloomberg School of Public Health, is one example of the global training programs launched to build capacity in low- and middle-income countries.[51]

Another key contribution the Bloomberg Initiative made to global tobacco control was the expansion of the Global Tobacco Surveillance System through the development of the Global Adult Tobacco Survey (GATS). GATS, launched in 2007, is a nationally representative household survey of adults (15 years old and older).[52] The survey enables countries to collect data on adult tobacco use and key tobacco control measures. Bloomberg Philanthropies committed more than $60 million to the CDC Foundation to support the development and implementation of GATS in its first five years.[53] Within this period, GATS was implemented in 14 countries where more than half of the world's smokers live, establishing a tobacco use baseline that represented four billion people.[54]

TABLE 5
Global Adult Tobacco Survey Results

Nation	Cigarette Smokers (%)		Nation	Cigarette Smokers (%)	
	Male	Female		Male	Female
Bangladesh	44.7	1.5	Russia	60.2	21.7
Brazil	21.6	13.1	Thailand	45.6	3.1
China	52.9	2.4	Turkey	47.9	15.2
Egypt	37.6	0.5	Ukraine	50.0	11.3
India	24.3	2.9	United Kingdom	22.8	20.6
Mexico	24.8	7.8	United States	24.0	16.2
Philippines	47.6	9.0	Uruguay	30.7	19.8
Poland	36.9	24.4	Vietnam	47.4	1.4

Global Adult Tobacco Survey. Data retrieved from http://www.theatlantic.com/health/archive/2012/08/tobacco-on-pace-to-kill-1-billion-people-this-century/261385/.

The Bloomberg Initiative was initially conceived in isolation from the broader FCTC process that was taking place globally at the time. At the beginning, there was little awareness or appreciation for the FCTC among the core leadership of the initiative. Consequently, instead of building on the momentum of the FCTC process or turning to the FCTC text, the Bloomberg Initiative sought a new paradigm for tobacco control in the form of MPOWER. MPOWER was a package of proven tobacco control strategies: "M" stood for monitoring tobacco use and the industry; "P," protecting non-smokers from exposure to secondhand tobacco smoke; "O," offering assistance to smokers who want to quit; "W," warning consumers of the health consequences of tobacco use; "E," enforcing bans on advertising, sponsorship, and promotion; and "R," raising tobacco taxes. The contents of MPOWER overlapped completely with that of the FCTC.

Although MPOWER did not have the buy-in and commitment from nearly every country in the world like the FCTC, it did have significant funding to support its implementation. Emphasis on MPOWER within WHO and other institutions (particularly those funded through the initiative) was immediate. Funding was provided to TFI, for example, to produce a biannual Global Tobacco Control Report (GTCR) that reviewed the status of tobacco control policy development in light of the MPOWER framework (not the FCTC).

The focus on MPOWER within TFI caused friction with the convention secretariat, who thought that WHO was turning its back on the treaty. TFI's call for countries to provide national reports for the GTCR, in addition to their reports to the COP, resulted in what the convention secretariat called "double reporting." TFI was eventually forced to use the FCTC country reports as the basis for the GTCR, although it continued to request additional information from countries that was not required in their official reports. Over time, WHO has finessed the divide between the FCTC and MPOWER (and TFI and the convention secretariat) by describing MPOWER as a tool to assist countries with implementing FCTC obligations.[55]

The influence of the Bloomberg Initiative was amplified by the near absence of other funding for FCTC implementation. The FCTC secretariat received $6 to $10 million per year to support the global implementation of the FCTC.[56] Per capita spending on tobacco control ranged from $1.30 per year in high-income countries to $0.011 in middle-income countries and $0.0003 in low-income countries.[57]

The funding the Bloomberg Initiative provided through grants and in-country capacity building provided viable career paths for many health professionals in low- and middle-income countries who would otherwise never have considered

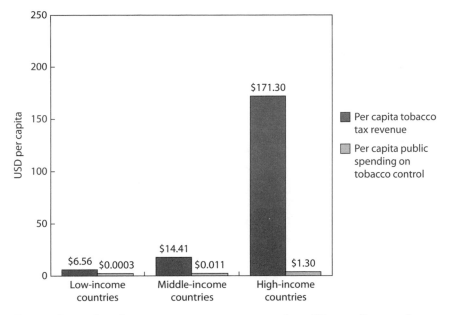

Figure 6. Per capita tobacco tax revenue versus per capita public spending on tobacco control, 2012. Data from the WHO Report on the Global Tobacco Epidemic, 2013

jobs in tobacco control. In five years, more than 7,000 public health professionals and 5,000 journalists from low- and middle-income countries received training in tobacco control that was supported by the initiative, and the numbers continued to climb.[58] The funds increased tobacco control advocates' ability to engage targeted governments and speed up policy adoption.

Arguably the most effective contribution the Bloomberg Initiative made to national tobacco policy change was the work carried out by the International Legal Consortium (ILC). The ILC was established by the Campaign for Tobacco-Free Kids and directed by Patricia Lambert, a South African human rights and labor lawyer. Before directing the ILC, Lambert served as legal advisor to the South African government and led the South African delegation during the FCTC negotiations. Lambert was a highly recognizable player in the FCTC negotiations and a symbol of the positive influence low- and middle-income countries (particularly from Africa) had on the fight for strong FCTC commitments. Lambert's team of six full-time lawyers and additional consultants traveled the world providing legal advice, revising draft legislation, training in-country lawyers, assisting in litigation, and helping combat industry interference. In its first five years, the ILC drafted or provided consultation in more than 60 countries.[59]

There is emerging evidence that the funding and activities carried out by the Bloomberg Initiative have significantly impacted global tobacco control networking and information sharing. A social network analysis of GLOBALink, for example, has shown that between 2006 and 2012 there was a significant shift in the centrality of the network toward the United States compared to during the FCTC process (1999–2005), when regional groupings became more pronounced and information sharing was more decentralized. The United States became the technological "gatekeeper" based on the resources (financing, expertise, access to influential decision-makers) that it brought to the network.[60] This change made sense given that most funds channeled to low- and middle-income countries through US-based organizations, including the Campaign for Tobacco-Free Kids (Washington, DC), the Johns Hopkins Bloomberg School of Public Health (Baltimore), the CDC Foundation (Atlanta), and the World Lung Foundation (New York City). The transition is highly ironic, though, because the United States is not party to the convention and has no official vote in the implementation and development of the treaty.

National Policy Implementation

As a public health treaty, the FCTC ultimately will be judged by how its contents are translated into effective national legislation and programs that reduce tobacco use and subsequently reduce tobacco-related diseases and death. Since the treaty entered into force, parties have made indisputable progress implementing the FCTC's provisions around the world. More than 75% of parties strengthened existing legislation or adopted new tobacco control laws after ratification.[61] There are numerous accounts of domestic policy change based wholly or in part on the FCTC text; these accounts began flowing in even before the FCTC was finalized.

Progress

Before the treaty's entry into force, countries began making policy changes to better align themselves with the treaty's goals. New Zealand, for example, passed a new law regarding the size of warning labels on tobacco products to bring itself in compliance with all articles in the FCTC. The Indian parliament responded to the FCTC process by passing the Cigarettes and Other Tobacco Products Act in 2003, and they approved India's ratification of the treaty. Malta altered its Tobacco Control Act and implemented the 2003 Smoking in Public Places Act in April 2004 to comply with its ratification of the FCTC in September 2003. The

Philippines' Tobacco Regulation Act of 2003, which limited the sale, sponsorship, and advertising of tobacco products, was a step toward the country's signing of the FCTC in October 2003. After its government signed the FCTC in March 2004, Uganda implemented a ban on public smoking despite the tobacco industry's profitable presence in the country.

In addition to these and many other qualitative reports of policy change resulting from the FCTC process and final text, there has been some limited quantitative research on the rate of policy change before, during, and after the treaty-making progress. An analysis of the passage of new laws regarding warning labels, smoking bans, and advertising restrictions revealed that the frequency of policy adoption in each case began to increase in 1998 and intensified between 2001 and 2003.[62] Moreover, the strength of the adopted policies shifted significantly throughout the 1998–2003 period, and the increase in adoption of tobacco control regulations was not limited to high-income countries. Since 2003, many of the earliest adopters of comprehensive tobacco control policy (e.g., Australia, Canada, Norway, and Singapore) have continued to innovate and have been joined by Brazil, South Africa, Turkey, Ukraine, and Uruguay. In fact, high-, middle-, and low-income countries experienced a significant rise in the adoption of tobacco control policies, with the greatest increase occurring in middle-income countries. Policy adoption also occurred in all regions, with the greatest rise occurring in Europe (likely a consequence of regional harmonization as opposed to FCTC obligations). Another study examining more than twenty years of data found that the passage of FCTC-compliant health warning label policies significantly accelerated after the FCTC entered into force, and that implementation of voluntary policies instituted by tobacco companies declined.[63]

A host of tools were also developed to assess the impact of the FCTC after it entered into force. Naturally, country reports to the COP were core instruments used to evaluate progress; however, they are based on self-reporting and have been criticized for lacking key information and rigorous review. Alternatively, the GTCR has tracked the passage of new MPOWER-relevant policies since its first edition in 2008. Although the GTCR is based on country reports to the COP, TFI also carried out an extensive review of the information to correctly categorize the strength of the policies and to collect additional data (e.g., tax data).

The 2013 GTCR, which was released 10 years after the adoption of the FCTC, found that more than 2.3 billion people—a third of the world's population—was protected at the time by at least one of the MPOWER measures at the highest recommended level of achievement.[64] Nearly 1.3 billion people were newly protected by at least one measure that had passed since 2008. The passage of complete

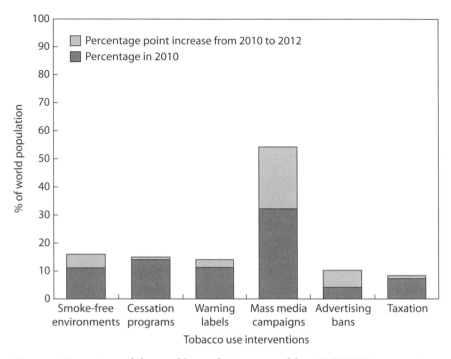

Figure 7. Percentage of the world population covered by MPOWER interventions against tobacco use in 2010 and the percentage-point increase from 2010 to 2012. Data from the WHO Report on the Global Tobacco Epidemic, 2013

public and workplace smoking bans were the most commonly established new measure: 32 countries passed complete smoking bans covering all workplaces, public places, and public transportation between 2007 and 2012, protecting nearly 900 million additional people.[65] New FCTC-compliant health warning labels on tobacco packaging were implemented in 20 countries, and complete bans on all tobacco advertising, promotion, and sponsorship were implemented in 16 countries, protecting more than half a billion people. Raising taxes to increase the price of tobacco products—the most effective tobacco control measure—remained rare. Only 14 countries and one territory increased their tax rates to the WHO-recommended level. Based on the policy changes reported in the GTCR between 2007 and 2010, one study concluded that the policy progress achieved in just three years would result in 7.5 million fewer smoking-related deaths by 2050.[66]

The International Tobacco Control Policy Evaluation Project (ITC) is yet another tool used to evaluate the implementation of the FCTC. The ITC Project is an international cohort study of tobacco use directed by Geoff Fong at the University of Waterloo in Canada. Its overall objective is to measure the psychosocial and behavioral impact of key national policies included in the FCTC. The study focuses on whether a given policy has its desired effect on the population as well as how and why those policy effects are achieved. By 2013, the ITC Project had been implemented in more than 20 countries, covering 50% of the world's population, 60% of the world's smokers, and 70% of the world's tobacco users.[67] In each country, researchers conducted prospective cohort surveys to assess the impact and identify the determinants of effective tobacco control policies related to health warning labels and package descriptors, smoke-free legislation, pricing and taxation of tobacco products, communication and education, cessation, and tobacco advertising and promotion. They follow up with the cohort every two years to measure changes over time.

The ITC Project has been instrumental in identifying the various impacts of policies on attitudes and behavioral change. Results from Thailand and Malaysia, for example, revealed that the larger and more informative Thai warnings on tobacco packaging were associated with higher levels of reactions that were predictive of quitting and stronger associations with subsequent quitting, demonstrating their potency.[68] The Project also has provided evidence of a high global demand for cessation, in line with FCTC article 14's guidelines on tobacco dependence and cessation, and it has provided data on the efficacy of quitline campaigns.[69] In addition, it revealed low rates of physician and other health professional advice to quit smoking in many countries. The results of the ITC surveys are shared through country and comparative reports provided by civil society to the COP.

The Global Youth Tobacco Survey (GYTS) and GATS are critical tools for evaluating the impact of the FCTC. Results from the GATS are meant to assist countries in the formulation, tracking, and implementation of effective tobacco control interventions, and countries are able to compare results of their survey to that of other countries. The first wave of the GATS between 2008 and 2010 provided a baseline by which to evaluate the impact of FCTC policy change on tobacco use. The survey generally found high rates of smoking in men, early initiation of smoking in women, and low quit ratios.[70] Subsequent waves of the GATS have provided powerful evidence of the impact effective tobacco control policies recommended by the FCTC and MPOWER can have on the reduction of smoking prevalence in a short period of time. In Uruguay, for example, between 2005 and 2011 the prevalence of tobacco use decreased annually by an estimated 3.3% (equivalent to 23% over 6 years). Uruguay's success is explored in detail in Part II of this book. Turkey, notably one of the Bloomberg Initiative's 15 priority countries, witnessed a 13% relative reduction in smoking prevalence between 2008 and 2012.[71]

Turkey's reduction in tobacco use followed an aggressive tobacco control program launched after the ratification of the FCTC in December 2004. Turkey was the third European country to go 100% smoke free in public places in 2008. A key element of Turkey's success has been its "whole-of-government" approach to tobacco control, led by former Prime Minister Recep Tayyip Erdoğan.[72] Driven by the Ministry of Health, a sophisticated system of intersectoral cooperation on policy initiatives was established within the Parliamentary Health Commission. In addition to the national coordination, a tobacco control board was established in every province. The membership of these boards consists of representatives of relevant public institutions, civil society organizations, and the local media. The boards have facilitated both the gathering of public support and supervision of the process.

Turkey's tobacco control success and corresponding decreases in tobacco use are all the more impressive given the large and powerful tobacco industry interests in the country, high prevalence of tobacco use (among the highest in Europe), and social acceptability of smoking when the program was launched. In such an environment, it was more critical than ever to engage a broad range of stakeholders in the decision-making and implementation of new laws. Prime Minister Erdoğan received the WHO director general's 2010 Special Recognition Award for Contribution to Global Tobacco Control for his personal commitment to tobacco control and his ability to bring diverse sectors together.

The Bloomberg Initiative's decision to launch the MPOWER package to advance optimal tobacco control policies in countries as opposed to sticking with the FCTC brand has made evaluation of the FCTC somewhat more complicated. The initiative expectedly claims credit for much of the significant tobacco control policy changes that have occurred since 2007. In evaluating its first five years of work, for example, the initiative pointed to the nearly 500% increase in the number of people protected from secondhand smoke in public places since its launch.[73] Although the initiative's financial and technical assistance often has been essential to push these policies forward, it is likely that the strong binding language on protection from passive smoking and comprehensive advertising bans in the FCTC also has been instrumental in the progressive adoption of such policies. In the end, the two tools reinforced each other and led to the strengthening of domestic tobacco control policies in numerous countries, thereby saving millions of lives.

Inaction

Whereas some parties have made very substantive progress since ratification of the treaty, others have failed to translate the treaty into meaningful domestic law or action. There are many reasons for inaction by such countries. The lack of substantial progress in Japan, China, and Germany, for example, is likely a consequence of the influential tobacco industry lobby in each of these countries. The domestic struggles in Germany and China are detailed in Part II of this book.

Lack of capacity and competing interests are also major challenges to the passage of tobacco control laws in many low- and middle-income countries. A case study of Ghana's delay in passing a tobacco control law in accordance with its FCTC obligations found that policymakers throughout the government were aware of the treaty and knew that Ghana needed to change its tobacco control laws to be compliant with its international commitments.[74] Through numerous interviews with policymakers, the study also revealed clear support for such tobacco control measures. This political support was evident when Ghana became the first West African country and thirty-ninth country in the world to ratify the FCTC.[75]

Many tobacco control advocates expected Ghana to continue to move quickly after ratification and pass a new law. A draft national tobacco control bill based on the FCTC was written in 2005, but was held up in the cabinet for years. Policymakers interviewed in the study stressed that tobacco control had not received the political attention or resources required to either enforce existing bans or pass a new law.[76] Given the strong support expressed by the policymakers, Ghana's inability to move on a tobacco control law likely was tied to industry influence on critical decision-makers. Although the policymakers interviewed for the study did not mention industry interference, NGO respondents stressed their ubiquitous presence and influence on the press.[77]

Ghana is typical of many low- and middle-income African countries in that its resources are limited, the prevalence of smoking remains low, and infectious disease epidemics such as HIV/AIDS and malaria continue to contribute significantly to the burden of disease. In this context, the tobacco industry is able to promote cheaper voluntary regulations, argue for lower taxes, and threaten expensive litigation against proposed innovative policy solutions.[78] Consequently, tobacco control remains largely in the form of directives and other uncoordinated legislative rules.

The situation in Ghana demonstrates how the FCTC process, although it has increased awareness among policymakers and clarified expectations for effective tobacco control, is not enough in countries with competing health priorities, limited resources, and the presence of transnational tobacco companies. International financial resources and political pressure are required to solidify political will, challenge the industry's presence, and move the tobacco control agenda forward.

There have been creative solutions to countering the influence of the tobacco industry in African countries. In Uganda, for example, a Tobacco Industry Monitoring (TIM) team was established after it became clear that the industry was interfering in the parliamentary process of passing a tobacco control bill that had been drafted in 2011.[79] The team comprises members of parliament (MPs) and tobacco control stakeholders from civil society. It monitors specific activities, including media and government activities. The team coordinator gathers intelligence from members each week and initiates any needed follow-up. In late 2013, an informant in parliament passed on information to the Uganda National Tobacco Control Association, which in turn informed the TIM that the industry had submitted a petition to the parliament's finance committee calling for a reduction of the Ministry of Finance's proposed excise tax on cigarettes from 44.5% in the 2013–2014 budget to 11.4%. With the support of WHO, the African Tobacco Control Alliance, and the Center for Tobacco Control in Africa, the TIM prepared a factsheet about the economic and public health benefits of a 44.5% increase.[80] The factsheet was given to ten MPs, who used its arguments to counter the industry's petition when the tax amendment bill was tabled in parliament.[81] In the end, the Ugandan parliament adopted the 45.5% increase.[82]

Implementation Challenges

In all countries, regardless of whether progress has already been made in implementing provisions of the FCTC, significant challenges to full implementation of the treaty remain. Although many of these challenges are specific to individual country settings and domestic realities, some are universal, including ongoing tobacco industry efforts to undermine the impact of the treaty, the rise of trade-related disputes between FCTC parties, and funding and coordination of the myriad of players now engaged in tobacco control efforts.

Tobacco Industry Opposition

In addition to the lobbying and influence exerted by the tobacco industry on national political processes, the transnational tobacco companies have also adopted broader global strategies to counter the impact of the FCTC on their business. Although the industry was divided on how to approach the negotiation of the FCTC, their failure to prevent its entry into force has resulted in the increasing alignment of their strategies.[83]

For example, the industry has increased investment in smokeless tobacco and production of other new "reduced-risk" products. The market share of smokeless tobacco has risen dramatically over the past few years in many countries, and the public health community is currently playing catch-up to understand the impact of these new products on health and tobacco control.[84] The popularity of electronic cigarettes is particularly troublesome. All major transnational tobacco companies now have substantial e-cigarette businesses. The FCTC did not anticipate such "non-tobacco" nicotine delivery systems, and these products have the potential to disrupt many aspects of traditional tobacco control and core FCTC policies, including tax, marketing, and product regulation.[85]

Another element of the new tobacco environment is the major effort underway by the top tobacco companies to remake their public image through new Corporate Social Responsibility (CSR) programs.[86] Transnational tobacco companies are increasingly recognizing the scientific literature on the health effects of active smoking, funding youth prevention programs, and, in some cases, even voicing support at the national level for ratification of the FCTC. They are also active in non-tobacco activities such as sponsoring the arts and supporting community programs. Companies may use CSR programs not just to enhance their public image, but also to gain access to politicians, influence agendas, and shape public health policy to best suit their own interests.

There is evidence that CSR programs have worked. By 2004, despite the entry into force of the FCTC, the stock value of Philip Morris/Altria completely recovered from losses incurred as a result of US litigation and stockholder distrust.[87] In 2004, BAT was awarded the Stakeholder Communication Award from the new PricewaterhouseCoopers Building Public Trust Awards.[88] The ability of the industry to translate their CSR activities into political influence underlined the need for parties to adopt strong implementation guidelines in relation to article 5.3 (protection of public health policies with respect to tobacco control from commercial and other vested interests).

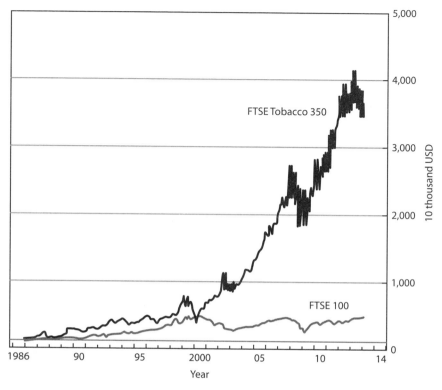

Figure 8. Tobacco industry stock, 1986–2014. Data from Bloomberg

International Trade Disputes

As predicted during the FCTC negotiations, WTO and other investment agreements have increasingly been used to frustrate national tobacco control initiatives in line with the objectives of the FCTC, and their use represents a key industry strategy to challenge FCTC implementation. Recent disputes under WTO law include the *United States–Clove Cigarettes* case in which the appellate body of the WTO held that parts of the US Family Smoking Prevention and Tobacco Control Act were inconsistent with WTO law.[89] In particular, the act's ban on clove but not menthol-flavored cigarettes was considered discrimination against products of Indonesian origin, and the United States was ordered to reopen its market to clove cigarettes (or ban menthol). In this case there was no consideration of the FCTC because neither the United States nor Indonesia was party to the treaty.

Another ongoing WTO case is *Australia–Plain Packaging*. In that dispute, a number of WTO members, many of whom are parties to the FCTC, are chal-

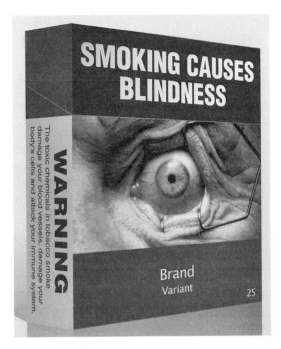

Figure 9. Australian plain package of cigarettes. © Commonwealth of Australia

lenging Australia's right to require plain packaging of tobacco products.[90] Various claims have been made against the packaging law, including that the measure unlawfully interferes with trademark rights and is more trade restrictive than necessary to protect health. This case raises the question of just how much authority any government has over the content and look of tobacco product packaging. The case also has implications for FCTC article 5.3 because the suing countries are clearly collaborating with the tobacco industry in their complaints and, therefore, are in violation of the convention.

In addition to these high-profile WTO disputes, tobacco companies have also recently brought claims against countries under other international investment agreements. For example, PMI has challenged Australia's plain packaging legislation under a bilateral investment treaty (BIT) between Australia and Hong Kong.[91] The company claims that plain packaging results in an expropriation of its property rights and is unfair and unreasonable. On similar grounds, the company has also challenged Uruguayan tobacco packaging and labeling measures under a BIT between that country and Switzerland.[92] In 2012, PMI lost a challenge claiming that Norway's bans on the display of tobacco products at the point of sale was illegal under the European Economic Area Agreement.[93] Those bans were found to be lawful by Oslo's district court because they are necessary to protect human health.

Tobacco control advocates have increasingly fought to exclude tobacco from all free trade and intellectual property agreements. However, efforts in 2013 to include an "exception clause" in the Trans-Pacific Partnership (TPP) hit a snag when the United States changed its position and refused to propose language excluding tobacco from the deal.[94] The TPP was a proposed trade agreement that would link the United States, Canada, Mexico, Japan, Australia, South Korea, Vietnam, and five other countries. Together the trade pact represented more than 40% of global trade.

Initially, the Obama administration favored a TPP provision exempting individual nations' tobacco regulations—such as those banning advertising or requiring warning labels—from legal attack because they are "non-tariff barriers" to the free flow of goods. However, at a public meeting in August 2013, the United States softened its position, proposing to include tobacco in an existing exemption for policies necessary to protect human life or health, and to require governments to consult before challenging each other's tobacco rules. Addressing the turnaround, the office of the US trade representative explained that the new stance came after resistance from members of Congress and a wide range of American stakeholders.[95] According to news reports, it appears to have been a result of major pushback from farm-state legislators, farm lobbies, and other interest groups that feared a tobacco exception would eventually expand to a health-related excuse for protectionism against many other products, such as unhealthy foods, non-alcoholic beverages, and alcohol.

Working with colleagues in the Southeast Asian Tobacco Control Alliance, tobacco control advocates were able to get Malaysia to counter the US proposal with demands that tobacco be excluded entirely from the negotiations.[96] The inability to resolve the tobacco carve-out language has threatened to derail the entire TPP process, with US tobacco control advocates uniting with other anti-trade coalitions to fight fast-track approval of the deal in Congress.

Many have argued that the Obama administration should cite the FCTC as grounds to treat tobacco differently than other products within trade law. Its unwillingness to do so thus far, and the overall rise of tobacco-related trade disputes, demonstrates the challenges that arise when multiple international legal regimes overlap. WHO's decision to use article 19 of its constitution to adopt binding conventions implied that it wanted health to be more seriously considered by governments and international institutions in global governing regimes.

However, unlike the conflict resolution mechanisms included in the global trade regime, the FCTC calls for disputes among two or more parties to be solved by "diplomatic channels." Therefore, all legally binding dispute resolution decisions are made through trade tribunals. Clearly, the tribunals established under BITs or the dispute settlement body of WTO does not understand or value health concerns as it does trade rules. This does not mean that they will not defend health interests, but that they will most likely do so with great deference to trade rules. The increasing number of conflicts, often with FCTC parties facing off against each other, raises the question of whether an international dispute settlement body for health-related issues should also be established.

Financial and Coordination Challenges

As mentioned previously, resources for tobacco control at the global and national levels are lacking, especially when compared to other global health priorities. Funding crises affecting WHO, for example, have reduced staff numbers and led to TFI's absorption into a general non-communicable disease prevention department.[97] Although philanthropic funding from Michael Bloomberg and Bill Gates has been helpful, more institutionalized and sustainable forms of financing will be needed in the long term.

There are multiple options still on the table for funding FCTC implementation, including requiring financial contributions from all parties according to their level of development, imposing new levies on repatriated tobacco revenue, and consolidating the administration of the FCTC by integrating WHO's tobacco control work into the FCTC secretariat. Other proposals include making mutual assistance programs conditional on the presence of an effective tobacco control program, or having donor countries reward innovative tobacco control measures developed in recipient countries that have measurable pre-agreed outcomes.[98] The FCA has also grown politically active in global processes related to the post-2015 FCTC development agenda and revised sustainable development goals in an effort to ensure that tobacco is identified as a development concern and funded through development programs. To date, less than two dozen countries have requested tobacco control support in their national development plans.[99]

The rise in trade disputes also represents an emerging financial challenge related to the implementation of the FCTC and effective tobacco control. Australia has already spent millions defending its plain packaging law, and Uruguay has accepted financial support from Bloomberg to defend its health warning laws. When announcing its intention to move forward with plain packaging, New Zealand announced that it anticipated having to spend up to $8 million to defend the law in court.[100] Most governments spend much less on tobacco control than the millions required to defend these laws in court, not to mention the potential losses incurred if governments lose the cases (Philip Morris is currently suing Uruguay for $2 billion).

Better coordination of FCTC implementation and financial assistance is needed to optimize what resources and existing global funds for tobacco control are available. Typical of other areas of global health governance, global tobacco control in the post-FCTC world is influenced by a plethora of groups, including WHO, ministries of health, WTO, NGOs, private foundations, and corporations (including health insurers, employers, pharmaceutical companies, technology companies, and wellness enterprises). The FCTC's short history has also shown the challenges that can arise from multi-stakeholder engagement. FCTC implementation, however, cannot be left to health ministries or departments of health alone. The failure to ratify the Protocol on Illicit Trade in Tobacco Products demonstrates the ongoing need to engage areas of government that deal with taxation, commerce, and customs, whereas the rise in trade disputes demonstrates the need for tobacco control to extend to foreign affairs, including international trade and foreign aid programs. The Turkish success story is a model for what can be achieved when a strong, multi-sectoral approach is taken to tobacco control.

Considerable progress was made implementing the FCTC during the decade following its adoption by the WHA. The COP and convention secretariat were established, and guidelines for implementation of the treaty were created. A reporting process and instrument were developed, with more than one hundred countries providing at least one publically available report. A single protocol on illicit trade was negotiated and adopted, although complications regarding its implementation resulted in countries' hesitancy to ratify.

Beyond this global institutional progress, the decade also contained a flurry of domestic tobacco control activity throughout the world. Much of this activity was the result of the financial investment and labor of the Bloomberg Initiative and the implementation of the MPOWER package. However, the FCTC provided the foundation on which to base this effort, empowered ministries of health to move forward with strong policy proposals, and imparted legitimacy to international involvement in domestic tobacco control policy processes.

There is no question that tobacco control policies are stronger on average today than they were when the FCTC was adopted. There is also more capability now to track the tobacco epidemic, and evidence is emerging that better policies are resulting in significant reductions in the prevalence of tobacco use in populations covered by those policies. FCTC implementation, however, is not even across countries or regions. Although some countries have been able to leverage the FCTC, others have seen little or no improvement in their domestic tobacco control situation in the post-FCTC period. Competing health priorities, financial crises, and industry interference have all challenged the effective implementation of the FCTC.

From the global perspective, there are many troubling signs for FCTC implementation as the treaty enters its second decade. The lack of sustainable financial mechanisms with which to support tobacco control programs in the long term offers a reality check to the progress driven largely thus far by philanthropic resources. Unresolved and growing conflicts between tobacco control and free trade pose significant challenges to fulfilling the FCTC's core objective of reducing disease and death caused by tobacco use. Finally, the complexity of addressing the tobacco issue globally and domestically challenges the basic premise that the FCTC is, in fact, a public health treaty. Although there is a clear need to retain the supremacy of health in the tobacco control fight, non-health partners are increasingly required to carry through with proposed policy solutions. But collaboration with other sectors, especially finance, trade, customs, and policing has proved difficult. These sectors have vastly different value systems and understandings of the way in which the world works. Their acceptance of the tobacco industry as a credible partner represents just one example of value conflicts that can complicate effective coordination of efforts.

There are numerous stories of tobacco control policy success and failure. Each one has elements that are universal and others that are specific to the unique national environment in which they took place. In the following chapters, I contrast the global FCTC story provided in the last three chapters with detailed domestic case studies. The case studies will illustrate the complexity involved in the passage of each one of the new policies mentioned in this chapter. There is nothing easy about tobacco control in any country, but the advances documented in this chapter provide enough evidence to claim that the FCTC negotiation process and its initial global implementation has been an irrefutable success.

PART TWO

NATIONAL EXPERIENCES

CHAPTER FIVE

The FCTC in Thailand

In Search of Solidarity

Throughout much of the twentieth century, tobacco use in Thailand was limited to the adult male population. In the early 1980s, for example, approximately 63% of Thai men smoked, whereas fewer than 5% of women smoked.[1] As was the case for many Asian countries, its high prevalence of male smoking and the unexploited female market made Thailand an attractive opportunity for transnational tobacco companies in search of new customers in the late 1980s. However, instead of quickly overtaking the domestic market as they had in numerous other low- and middle-income countries in Latin America, Eastern Europe, and Asia, transnational tobacco companies faced fierce and effective opposition to their foray into Thailand.

Working closely with international tobacco control advocates, the Thai government fought (unsuccessfully) against the US trade office to keep transnational tobacco companies out of the country. Once forced to open its domestic market, Thailand passed comprehensive tobacco control legislation in the early 1990s to blunt the impact of the transnational tobacco companies. Consequently, smoking prevalence in Thailand fell steadily from 59.3% for males and 5% in females in 1991 to 40.5% and 2% in 2009, respectively: an aggregate 35% drop over 18 years.[2] Despite massive transnational tobacco investment and lobbying, Thailand was able to achieve this significant reduction in the number of men who smoke while also keeping female smoking rates low.

The history of tobacco control in Thailand in the late 1980s and 1990s is in many ways symbolic of the underlying rationale for the Framework Convention on Tobacco Control. Thailand provided the model of a middle-income country joining high-income advocates in the fight against the tobacco industry, and it delivered evidence of the effectiveness of comprehensive tobacco control within a developing country context.

Thai tobacco control advocates were vocal supporters of the FCTC from its inception. At the start of the FCTC process, Thai advocates argued that international collaboration through the FCTC was required to combat transnational forces that were negatively impacting their tobacco control efforts, including cross-border marketing and illicit trade. Thai advocates also saw the FCTC as an instrument through which to promote international solidarity against the transnational tobacco industry. Through close collaboration between Thai governmental and non-governmental representatives, Thailand became a leader in efforts to develop a strong treaty and resist challenges to the FCTC by the Big Four (Japan, Germany, United States, and China). However, Thai officials and tobacco control advocates faced numerous challenges to obtaining the treaty that they desired because of their progressive objectives and their relatively weak political position in the international system.

As pledged, Thai tobacco control advocates have successfully used the treaty text to advocate for new legislation and further strengthen the country's overall tobacco control program since the FCTC entered into force in Thailand in February 2005. Thai tobacco control advocates have also become effective international leaders, sharing their expertise with other countries in the Southeast Asian region and beyond. Tobacco control in Thailand has often been defined by complex sociocultural, deeply personal, and at times corrupt dynamics. The process, however, through which tobacco control advocates have been able to achieve success, including identifying best practices from abroad, translating these practices to their domestic environment, and using shrewd tactics to obtain the political support needed to pass and implement new laws, provides a powerful example to advocates around the world looking to bring change to their domestic tobacco control environment.

Pre-FCTC Thailand

Descriptions of Thailand's involvement in tobacco control often begin with the Thai tobacco case in the General Agreement on Tariffs and Trade (GATT) in 1989–1990. However, the struggle for tobacco control in Thailand began long before as a small domestic civil society movement supported by a number of medical associations. In 1974, the Thai Medical Association successfully petitioned the government to print health warnings on cigarette packages.[3] In 1980, the Thai Ministry of Health partnered with the Thai Thoracic Association, the Thai Anti-Tuberculosis Association, and the Thai Heart Association on a series of public education programs on the dangers of smoking, which resulted in the Thai tobacco monopoly further strengthening health warnings on tobacco packages.[4] In 1982, the Thai Ministry of Public Health (MOPH) partnered with the World Health Organization to hold the First National Conference on Tobacco or

Health, which resulted in the ministry's inclusion of tobacco as a health issue in its non-communicable disease division (although no resources were allocated specifically for tobacco).[5]

The early tobacco control movement in Thailand received a major boost in 1986 when the Thai Anti-Smoking Campaign Project (TASCP) was formed within the Folk Doctor Foundation with funding from a respected university professor and opinion leader, Dr. Prawase Wasi. Key individuals involved with the launch of the TASCP were Professor Athasit Vejjajiva, then dean of Ramathidobi Hospital and a member of the faculty of medicine at Mahidol University, and Prakit Vateesatokit, then chairman of the Department of Medicine at Mahidol University. Bungon Rittiphakdee, then a staff member at the Folk Doctor Foundation, was put in charge of running the daily operations of the project.[6] All three individuals would become leaders of the Thai tobacco control movement for decades to come. The TASCP was renamed Action on Smoking and Health, or ASH Thailand, in 1996.

The TASCP initially focused exclusively on promoting knowledge about the health effects of tobacco use, and its members lacked appreciation for the importance of a comprehensive legislative strategy. The sixth World Conference on Tobacco or Health (WCTOH) in 1987 provided one of the first opportunities for Thai advocates to learn about legislative approaches to control tobacco in other countries. They heard firsthand from top international experts such as Judith Mackay of the Asian Tobacco Consultancy, Richard Doll and Richard Peto from Oxford University, and Greg Connolly from the Massachusetts Department of Health.[7] Shortly thereafter, Richard Peto visited Thailand and, based on his research, projected that one million Thai children could be saved from cigarette smoke–related deaths if Thailand enacted comprehensive tobacco control legislation.[8]

It was at this same time that the government-owned Thai Tobacco Monopoly (TTM) requested funds from the Thai government to build a new, more efficient tobacco factory. The TTM was "fat and extremely uncompetitive," as was typical of government monopolies, and struggled to compete with the increasing (illegal) presence of transnational companies.[9] The request for an upgraded factory was initially approved, and the TASCP responded by fueling major media protests, this time calling for a comprehensive tobacco control plan.[10] In an effort to seize the moral high ground and attract positive media attention, then Prime Minister General Prem Tinsulanonda backed down from supporting the development of a new factory for the TTM (although it was eventually built) and publicly stated that it was not right for the government to earn income from such an inappropriate source.[11] In addition, he instructed the MOPH to draft a new comprehensive plan for tobacco control.

Dr. Hatai Chitanondh, deputy director of the MOPH's Department of Medical Services, was responsible for drafting the comprehensive plan. Besides facilitating an alliance between the MOPH and TASCP, Dr. Chitanondh would help determine the course of Thai tobacco control over the next decade and a half. At the time, he was a relatively new convert to the tobacco control movement; in fact, when he was appointed deputy director (and thus became responsible for the National Cancer Institute in Thailand) he was still a pipe smoker.[12] Dr. Chitanondh first became aware that Thailand had not implemented WHO-recommended tobacco control policies when he read a WHO paper on the growing tobacco epidemic in the mid-1980s. He immediately began researching the issue of tobacco control and writing a comprehensive review of tobacco use in Thailand.[13] By the time Dr. Chitanondh was formally instructed to draft a national tobacco control plan, he was well educated on tobacco control legislative approaches used in other countries. He specifically turned to legislation from Sweden, Australia, and Canada for ideas in developing the Thai plan.[14] In April 1988, the MOPH presented the tobacco control plan written by Dr. Chitanondh to the Thai cabinet. The cabinet unanimously passed the plan.

The new national tobacco control plan included a comprehensive advertising ban, which was initially welcomed by the TTM. In the late 1980s, Thailand was suddenly awash with cigarette advertisements for illegal international brands. Between January 1988 and February 1989, before the Thai market opened itself to international tobacco products, the transnational tobacco companies spent well over 17,085,100 Baht ($500,000) on advertising in Thailand.[15] As a result of this international advertising campaign, the TTM was forced to greatly increase its own advertising expenditures and for a short period engaged in an advertising war with foreign companies.[16] The advertising ban let them off the hook.

In December 1988, the TTM began protesting to the government that the transnational tobacco companies were still advertising despite the ban. The foreign companies responded that the cabinet prohibition was an executive order, not a law, and did not have to be followed by the private sector.[17] The cabinet instructed the Consumer Protection Board to find a new means of stopping cigarette advertising by law. In February 1989, the board added tobacco to the list of regulated products that could not be advertised under the 1979 Consumer Protection Act. The international companies were given one month to dismantle and remove all of their billboards and advertisements.[18]

Despite the advertising presence of the international tobacco control companies, they were not allowed to formally operate in Thailand. Since the end of the Second World War, tobacco production and manufacturing in Thailand was completely controlled by the TTM. The Thai Ministry of Finance formally proposed opening the market to foreign cigarettes in March 1989. Tobacco control advocates worked with a number of other groups to oppose entry of the international tobacco companies into the Thai market. The anti-entry alliance launched an effective media campaign against the proposal, and the government grew increasingly unwilling to side with tobacco interests. As a result of this pressure, the Ministry of Finance was forced to withdraw its proposal to open the Thai cigarette market to foreign companies.[19]

Thailand versus US GATT Case

For many people in Thailand, especially those from the public health and medical sectors, it appeared in early 1989 that they had won the war against the transnational tobacco companies. The Thai market was closed to international tobacco products, advertising of all cigarette products was banned, and the government appeared dedicated to tobacco control. It came as a shock when, two months after the Ministry of Finance withdrew its proposal to open the Thai market, the news media reported that the US trade office was investigating Thailand under chapter 301 of the 1974 US Trade Act. Section 301 authorizes the US president to take all appropriate action, including retaliation, to remove any act, policy, or practice of a foreign government that violates an international trade agreement or is unjustified, unreasonable, or discriminatory, and that burdens or restricts US commerce. Section 301 cases can be self-initiated by the United States Trade Representative (USTR) or as the result of a petition filed by a firm or industry group, in this case the US tobacco companies. If the USTR initiates a section 301 investigation, it must seek to negotiate a settlement with the foreign country in the form of compensation or elimination of the trade barrier. For cases involving trade agreements, the USTR is required to request formal dispute proceedings as stipulated in the agreements.

According to Dr. Prakit Vateesatokit,[20] before 1989 neither Thai policymakers nor the medical professionals advocating for tobacco control had any idea who the international tobacco companies were, and they were much less aware of the companies' aggressive tactics to open tobacco markets elsewhere in Asia. Dr. Vateesatokit said, "While we knew Marlboro cigarettes, neither I nor anyone else working in tobacco control in Thailand had ever heard of Philip Morris."[21] Although the US investigation came as a surprise to him and many others in Thailand, it was not surprising to members of the international tobacco control community who had witnessed as Japan, Taiwan, and Korea all reluctantly gave in to US pressure on cigarette trade under chapter 301. These international tobacco control advocates saw Thailand as the last step the industry needed to take to open the entire Asian market and as a potential test case to stand up to the United States in the name of public health.[22] The John Tung Foundation, a tobacco control NGO in Taipei, Taiwan, invited Drs. Vateesatokit and Chitanondh to a meeting to decide on a strategy for confronting the USTR. Other invitees included Greg Connolly from the Massachusetts Department of Health, Richard Daynard from Northeastern University in Boston, and Terry Pechacek from the US National Cancer Institute, as well as tobacco control advocates from Japan, Korea, and Taiwan.[23] At the Taipei meeting, Dr. Connolly first suggested negotiating with the USTR from the perspective of health rather than trade.[24]

During two official negotiating sessions between the Thai and US governments, the United States insisted that Thailand lift its advertising ban, repeal its import tax on tobacco products, and allow foreign companies to set up their own tobacco distribution system within Thailand—none of which the Thais were prepared to do. Consequently, the USTR referred the dispute to a GATT panel. Several rounds of testimony before the GATT panel were held in 1990 in Geneva, Switzerland. As previously suggested by Dr. Connolly, Thailand defended its position based on its public health rationale. Both Drs. Vateesatokit and Chitanondh were members of the Thai committee to GATT, and Dr. Connolly represented WHO in support of Thailand's position. The United States was supported by the European Union.

The GATT dispute, which occurred under General Chunhawan's coalition government, provided the first platform on which various ministries in the Thai government worked together on the tobacco issue—something that didn't occur in many other countries until the FCTC negotiations a decade later.

On September 25, 1990, the GATT panel ruled that Thailand's import ban was contrary to trade provisions and that Thailand should open its market to foreign cigarettes.[25] However, the panel also ruled that Thailand could maintain its advertising ban and introduce tobacco control policies as long as they applied equally to both domestic and foreign products. For many in Thailand, especially those in the Ministry of Commerce, the GATT ruling was seen as an embarrassing defeat to the United States. However, the nuanced ruling provided an opportunity for Thai policymakers to make it clear that they were still in control of their domestic tobacco market. The opportune time to introduce tobacco control legislation had arrived.

Legislation

While the GATT process was underway, the law subcommittee of the National Committee for the Control of Tobacco Use met often to draft a Tobacco Products Control Act. Although the bill previously had faced numerous challenges, the GATT ruling provided additional momentum for its adoption given the general sentiment that new legislation would counteract the image of Thailand having lost to the United States. On October 9, 1990, the cabinet approved the Ministry of Commerce's proposal to open up the Thai market to foreign cigarettes as instructed by GATT, and on the same day, the cabinet requested from the MOPH a copy of the draft tobacco control bill. Less than a week later, on October 15, 1990, the cabinet approved in principle the draft Tobacco Products Control Act and established the Office for Tobacco Consumption Control within the MOPH.[26]

In February 1991, a military coup saw Chatichai Choonhavan's government replaced by an unelected government with a cabinet of technocrats led by former diplomat Anand Panyarachun. In this new political scenario, tobacco control advocates had direct access to new Deputy Health Minister Athasit Vejjajiva, one of the founders of TASCP, former dean of the Ramathidobi Hospital, and close personal confidant of Dr. Vateesatokit.[27] On March 21, 1991, Dr. Chitanondh sent Deputy Health Minister Vejjajiva a personal letter with a draft ministerial order to establish a new drafting committee with himself as chair and Dr. Vateesatokit as a member. Deputy Health Minister Vejjajiva promptly appointed the new committee and charged them with revising and completing the draft Tobacco Products Control Act and drafting a new National Health Promotion Act.[28] In June 1991, the committee completed its work and the draft texts were forwarded to the public health minister before proposal to the cabinet.

After waiting for months for the texts to be considered, the two bills were finally passed by the cabinet and forwarded to the National Assembly in February 1992. Scandalous stories of industry infiltration and last-minute deals in the legislative committee followed. Previously confidential tobacco industry documents now confirm that the deputy prime minister, for example, was a key ally of the transnational tobacco companies and was instrumental in delaying consideration of the bills and building a strong coalition of lawmakers in opposition to the proposed laws.[29] Tobacco control advocates, however, used their close ties to the government leadership and intense media coverage to uncover the transnational companies' influence on Thai policymaking. Consequently, the final texts of the Thai Tobacco Products Control Act and the Non-Smokers' Health Protection Act were passed together by the Thai General Assembly on March 13, 1992.[30]

The 1992 legislation was among the most comprehensive tobacco control legislation in place anywhere in the world. The Tobacco Products Control Act banned all forms of cigarette advertising, cigarette promotions and free samples, and advertising of other products in which a cigarette brand is part of the logo. Sales of cigarettes were also prohibited to individuals younger than 18 years old, and cigarette vending machines were banned. Cigarette manufacturers were required to devote at least 35% of total package space to a black-and-white health warning. Manufacturers and importers of tobacco products were also obliged to inform the MOPH of the composition of their products before they could be sold.[31] Such an ingredient disclosure policy was only in place at the time in one other country in the world: Canada. The Non-Smokers' Health Promotion Act essentially banned smoking in all public buildings.[32]

Implementation and Enforcement

After the end of the Panyarachun government, the tobacco multinationals sought to win back lost territory, and the MOPH struggled to effectively implement the new laws. The transnational tobacco companies were most concerned with the requirement of the Tobacco Products Control Act that cigarette firms disclose the ingredients of their products.[33] The act itself did not specify requirements for ingredient disclosure, but rather required that a ministerial regulation be subsequently developed. The transnational tobacco companies sought to obstruct or delay the development of the ministerial regulation by all possible means.

The industry's commitment to resisting Thailand ingredient legislation came from a fear of a domino effect regionally and globally.[34] Industry documents warned of "a dangerous precedent which could affect us in other markets" and "could carry serious global repercussions."[35] British American Tobacco's Andrew Leung argued that:

> It sets a real bad example for other Asia-Pacific markets to follow. Although Canada is the first one to require ingredient disclosure, Asia-Pacific markets usually regard Canada as a low profile developed Western country that is different from them. Thailand now comes up with a more stringent set of requirements, other Asia-Pacific markets will definitely look into the issue and they will be under pressure from anti-smoking activists to follow suit.[36]

Throughout 1992 and 1993, the transnational tobacco companies were successful in stalling the drafting of a regulation on ingredient disclosure. Their success largely depended on the elected politicians who took turns assuming control of the MOPH, which changed hands nine times between 1992 and 1998.[37] Industry documents reflect structural corruption characteristic of Thai politics during this period.[38] For example, a BAT note from a February 1993 meeting with then Minister of Health Kaewattana Boonphan concludes "the only means of negotiation with politicians is dollar and cent."[39]

The transnationals' position in relation to ingredient disclosure became more difficult in 1994 after New Zealand required public disclosure of ingredient lists under its freedom of information legislation.[40] Finally, in 1995, Minister of Health Arthit Ourairat, a technocrat friendly with tobacco control advocates, pushed the regulation through in the last cabinet meeting of his government for the year.[41] Even then, it took two more years before the regulation was signed into law by Minister of Public Health Montri Pongpanich (who, industry documents allege, requested $5 million not to sign).[42]

After six years of delay, the ingredient disclosure law came into effect in late 1998. However, largely under pressure from embassies and trade representatives of the transnational tobacco companies' home governments in the United States, United Kingdom, and Japan, the MOPH announced that disclosures would be kept confidential.[43] Consequently, the impact of the ingredient disclosure law was greatly reduced and advocates have since argued that the confidential disclosures are largely meaningless.

Other policies in the Tobacco Products Control Act were also difficult to implement. The act's ban on advertising and promotion, for example, provided an ongoing point of contention between the transnational companies and the Thai government. Having failed to gain the right to advertise, foreign cigarette companies instead tried to circumvent the law. Various forms of indirect advertisements of foreign cigarettes continued after the law was passed.[44] Camel Trophy (an off-road car race sponsored by Japan Tobacco International) and Marlboro Classic goods, as well as bumper stickers with foreign cigarette logos, were widely available.[45] The transnational tobacco companies also increasingly engaged in philanthropy by sponsoring arts, sport, and cultural activities.[46]

Technically speaking, the MOPH was (and continues to be) responsible for enforcement of the advertising ban. However, the ministry was not skilled in carrying out such work and had very little resources for it. The Thai Health Promotion Institute, a non-governmental organization (NGO) set up by Dr. Chitanondh after his retirement from the MOPH, became the main monitoring force for advertising and promotion.[47] The institute itself has no authority in law enforcement, but it has provided numerous notifications of violations to the Institute of Tobacco Consumption Control at the Department of Medical Services (the office formally charged with enforcement).[48] Although there have been no official reports of advertising violations recorded by the MOPH, in a few cases suppression of the tobacco industry's promotional activities has been successful thanks to the Thai Health Promotion Institute's vigilance and strong media advocacy.[49]

The Tobacco Products Control Act's ban on sales to people younger than 18 years old was another challenge to implement. A 1996 purchase survey showed that 97% of 15-year-olds who tried to purchase cigarettes in Thailand were successful.[50] Unlike in Europe or the United States, where cigarettes are sold in stores and can be kept behind the counter or in locked cabinets, cigarettes in Thailand (as in most low- and middle-income countries) are often sold on the street and in small shops. Single cigarettes are also sold, making it even more difficult to keep them out of the hands of teenagers and children.

There were also challenges to enforcing the initial ban on smoking in public places. A 1997 report revealed that during the National Health Promotion Bill's first five years, there was no record of fines for smoking in prohibited areas.[51] However, this is not to say that the law was completely ignored. Strong education programs and media attention did result in high public compliance, and Thai society, at least in Bangkok, was widely considered to be anti-smoking prior to ratification of the FCTC.[52]

Taxation

In addition to its strong tobacco control laws, Thailand was also successful at passing tobacco taxation before 2000. A tobacco tax was first passed in 1993. The Thai government earned more than 40 billion Baht ($1 billion) in additional revenue through cigarette tax increases between 1992 and 1999, and smoking prevalence fell from 26.3% to 20.5% during this time.[53] Moreover, it was estimated that increases in excise tax caused up to 200,000 young smokers to quit in the mid-1990s alone.[54] Between 1994 and 2003 the tax was increased six additional times, and in 2003 it comprised 75% of the retail price of cigarettes.[55]

Not only were tobacco taxes successfully implemented and raised, but they were also successfully earmarked for health promotion. When advocates first pressed for an excise tax in 1993, no request for money for tobacco control was made at the time to avoid accusations of self-interest. In 1996, Supakorn Buasia, then deputy director of the Health Systems Research Institute, and Dr. Vateesatokit took advantage of a visit by Rhonda Galbally, the chief executive officer of Australia's Victorian Health Promotion Foundation (VicHealth), to press the issue of earmarking tobacco taxes for tobacco prevention.[56] VicHealth is a statutory autonomous organization in Australia that has been funded by a dedicated to-bacco tax since 1987. The two accompanied Dr. Galbally to a meeting with the minister of finance, who, as part of the government's decentralization policy, had already begun to consider the idea of using tax revenues for a health insurance scheme and for health promotion. After the meeting and at the request of the minister of finance, a small Thai delegation went to Australia to examine how VicHealth used a dedicated tax to promote health. The delegation then prepared draft legislation that set up the Health Promotion Office as an autonomous agency within the prime minister's office that was funded by a dedicated tax of 2.5% to 3% of the tobacco tax. The Health Promotion Bill was sent to the cabinet for approval in late 1996.[57]

Progress on the idea of a ThaiHealth Promotion Foundation funded by to-bacco taxes halted in 1997 after the Asian financial crisis. Work on the Health Promotion Bill did not resurface until 1999, when, by coincidence, the deputy minister of finance was admitted to Ramathibodi Hospital as a patient. Dr. Prakit Vathesatogkit, then dean of the university hospital, visited the deputy minister and secured his promise to help move the Health Promotion Bill forward. Over the following two years, the tobacco tax bill was heavily debated but subsequently passed by the Thai Senate on September 26, 2001. Final support for the bill was gained after the election of a new government that included universal health coverage in its agenda. The Health Promotion Office, already formed in 2000, now had significant funding ($35 million per year) and became the ThaiHealth Promotion Foundation (ThaiHealth).

Since 2001, there has been much concern and political controversy over how the budget of ThaiHealth should be spent, with many arguing that funds could be used for other, more urgent purposes. Dr. Abhisit Vejjajiva's appointment as chairman of the board was crucial in defending the activities of the Health Promotion Office, and under his leadership, tobacco control efforts grew dramatically. The appointment of Supakorn Buasia as director of ThaiHealth, noted above as a critical player in getting the tobacco tax on the agenda, also greatly benefited the organization and tobacco control interests in Thailand. The high level of credibility afforded both individuals, as well as their political influence, has been critical in defending the ThaiHealth budget. Both have had to withstand aggressive personal attacks directed at the use of funds for health promotion.

Thailand and the FCTC Process

Although much progress had been achieved in Thailand before the launch of the FCTC process, it was still difficult to say that the Thai government was solidly in favor of tobacco control. At every turn, tobacco control advocates faced strong tobacco industry lobbying and influence, and they used personal favors and political maneuvering to push their bills through. During the previous decade, the close collaboration established between the different ministries during the GATT case had fallen apart. Moreover, Thailand's experience with increasingly reduced tariffs as a result of the Asian Free Trade Agreement (AFTA), cross-border marketing and internet sales, and illicit trade all pointed to its inability to single-handedly control tobacco within its borders. Thus, from the start, Thai MOPH officials and advocates looked to the FCTC as a platform to further institutionalize tobacco control in Thailand and gain international partners in its efforts to monitor and withstand tobacco industry pressure.

Process Leadership

Dr. Hatai Chitanondh was appointed as the permanent chair of the official Thai delegation to the Intergovernmental Negotiating Bodies (INBs). In this role, he took on multiple leadership positions throughout the development of the FCTC, including chairing INB working group 1. Working group 1 was responsible for negotiating a number of the most significant issues addressed by the FCTC, including issues particularly key to Thailand, such as research, regulation of tobacco product disclosure, sales to youth, packaging and labeling, treatment of tobacco dependence, exposure to tobacco smoke, regulation of contents of tobacco products, and advertising, promotion, and sponsorship.

To support the FCTC process, Thailand also partnered with WHO to host multiple meetings to facilitate the negotiations, including the second Intersessional Meeting for Member States in the Association of Southeast Asian Nations, which was held before INB5 in Bangkok in 2002 and chaired by Thailand. Ten ASEAN countries and seven NGOs reviewed the chair's proposed text and endorsed the Bangkok Declaration on Tobacco Control, which promoted an ASEAN response to the tobacco epidemic. It was agreed at this meeting that, for those items on which consensus was reached, interventions at INB5 would be presented as ASEAN positions.[58] Thailand also played a lead role in several other working groups, including chairing the Working Group on Health and Education Issues after INB1.

Negotiating Positions

Going into the FCTC negotiations, Thai delegates and advocates called for inclusion of tobacco control gold standards in the treaty. These standards included supporting measures that would effectively eradicate tobacco smuggling, a global ban on tobacco advertising and sponsorship, the elimination of duty-free sales of tobacco products, the harmonization of taxes on tobacco products at the international level, the exemption of tobacco products from reduced taxation under regional free-trade agreements, mandatory testing and reporting of toxic constituents, and the establishment of mechanisms for information sharing.

Thailand's progressive positions were very much in line with those of the Framework Convention Alliance and other tobacco control NGOs, and it provided leadership from the beginning in terms of civil society participation in the FCTC process. As described in Chapter 3, Thailand joined Canada at INB1 in successfully securing civil society participation in the process. However, Thailand's impact on non-governmental participation in the FCTC went far beyond the official delegation's support for NGO participation in the INBs. The blurred lines between members of Thailand's official delegation and the Action on Smoking and Health (ASH) membership meant that Thai advocates had a direct line to official Thai negotiating positions, which provided an avenue for them to insert specific language into the negotiations. The Thai delegation actively participated in countless civil society briefings held during the negotiations. The intimacy of the relationship between organizations led some to claim that Thai delegates were operating on behalf of the NGOs and were not representative of the official Thai government positions.

During the negotiations, Thailand was perhaps most notorious for its leadership in challenging the United States and Japan's efforts to prioritize trade during the negotiations. Thailand's past experience with GATT provided the foundation for its global leadership on the issue. Thailand pushed for specific language placing health over trade, arguing "if the Framework Convention does not explicitly state that its public health provisions are to take priority when they conflict with trade rules, it would allow the industry to challenge other provisions of the Convention as trade violations."[59] After failing to get other, particularly high-income countries, to join the fight, Dr. Chitanondh personally intervened as chair. However, as highlighted in Chapter 3, Thailand failed in its effort to gain explicit language prioritizing health over trade, and the ambiguous language of the final treaty text remains a major point of debate. Since the FCTC's entry into force, the

rise of trade litigation against countries for their domestic tobacco control policies underlines Thailand's early understanding of the implications of this text.

Thailand also stood up to efforts to add reservations to the final treaty. Dr.
Chitanondh used the unpopularity of the US military buildup in Iraq as a way of
gaining political support from other countries to resist US pressure to add reservations. In this case, Thailand was able to overcome its relatively weak political
position to assure the strength and integrity of the treaty.

Civil Society

Although present from the beginning, non-governmental Thai advocates began
to take on more and more international leadership as the FCTC process continued. For example, ASH Thailand was a founding member of the FCA, and FCA
global headquarters were based in Bangkok at the ASH Thailand offices for many
years. In 2001, with support from the Rockefeller Foundation, ASH Thailand
established the Southeast Asian Tobacco Control Alliance (SEATCA). SEATCA
supported FCTC-related activities in neighboring countries, including holding
research and advocacy training workshops, carrying out multi-country research,
and disseminating advocacy materials. SEATCA, directed by longstanding Thai
tobacco control advocate Bungon Ritthiphakdee, became an invaluable resource
in the region and further established Thailand as a regional and global tobacco
control leader. Ritthiphakdee was awarded the WHO Director General Award on
Tobacco Control in the midst of the FCTC negotiations in 2001 for her leadership in the establishment of SEATCA.

Interestingly, Thai advocates, including Ritthiphakdee, discount their influence on the FCTC negotiations. Ritthiphakdee points to language challenges and
the inability to passionately communicate in English as one cause for their occasional marginalization. The role of Thailand as a relatively small, middle-income
country may have also marginalized their influence in the formal international
system.

FCTC Ratification

Thailand ratified the FCTC on November 8, 2004, making it one of the first forty
countries to do so. The fact that Thailand already had the required laws in place,
as well as its reputation as a global leader in tobacco control, made ratification
an easy sell to policymakers. The treaty entered into force on February 28, 2005.
Since ratification, Thailand has remained engaged in the FCTC process, hosting

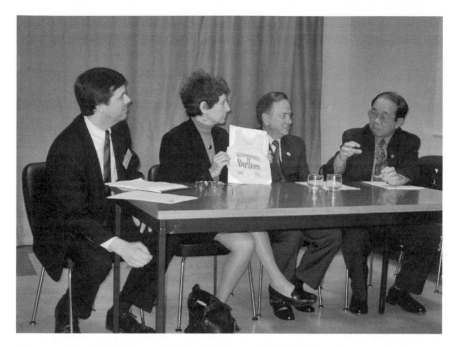

Figure 10. Dr. Hatai Chitanondh (far right) at an NGO briefing. Framework Convention Alliance

the second Conference of Parties in Bangkok from June 30 to July 6, 2007. At this meeting, Dr. Chitanondh was elected COP president in recognition of his leadership role throughout the FCTC process. Reflecting Thailand's experience, this COP focused especially on article 5.3 (industry interference) and established a working group to develop guidelines for country implementation of treaty obligations in relation to interacting with and monitoring the tobacco industry. Thailand was a member of a study group on alternative crops established by the first session of the COP, and it also actively participated in the negotiations of the FCTC protocol on illicit trade. Illicit trade was a topic of concern for Thailand from the beginning of the FCTC process, and it has continued to push for strong measures in this area, particularly concerning technical cooperation and capacity building, which it argued was essential to attract enough countries to participate.

Post-FCTC Tobacco Control in Thailand

At the time of ratification, Thailand was almost entirely compliant with the treaty text. Regardless, Thai advocates have continued to push for new tobacco control legislation to bring the country more in line with the objectives of the convention. Thai advocates have repeatedly argued that the FCTC is a guideline, and that they are committed to ensuring that Thailand's laws go well beyond the basic requirements of the treaty. In the eight years since ratification, they have had repeated successes in this regard.

Legislation

A flurry of tobacco control laws, particularly in regard to advertising, second-hand smoke, and package and labeling, have been passed in Thailand since it ratified the FCTC. In 2005, Thailand closed a loophole in its advertising law that banned point-of-sale advertising and brought it in compliance with FCTC article 13. Consequently, all tobacco displays in the country must be kept out of sight. In February 2008, the national smoking ban was extended to include entertainment outlets, open-air markets, restaurants, and bars, and in 2010, smoking was banned in all indoor public places. Recent studies suggest that the household setting is now one of the most significant sources of secondhand smoke exposure in the Thai population, especially for children and youth, which challenges the reach of traditional legislative approaches. In 2008 and 2009, Thailand passed policies allocating substantial funding for a national quitline (FCTC article 14) and increasing taxes (FCTC article 6). Although Thailand was now in compliance with FCTC article 14 (tobacco dependence and cessation), the usage rates of quitlines, cessation clinics, and nicotine-replacement therapy (NRT) were still low among attempted quitters (0.7%, 1.5%, and 2.5%, respectively), whereas unassisted cessation rate by doctor counseling ranged from 10% to 20%.[60]

In 2010, the National Committee for the Control of Tobacco Use (NCCTU) developed a National Strategic Plan for Tobacco Control that incorporated many suggested measures contained in the FCTC. The plan was not formally adopted by the Thai cabinet until June 2012, after the Thai 2011 GATS showed a 1% increase in smoking prevalence among adult males (from 45.6% to 46.6%) between 2009 and 2011.[61] This was the first time in 20 years that smoking prevalence in Thailand showed any increase, prompting the Thai cabinet to approve the Ministry of Health's National Strategic Plan for Tobacco Control and, on August 21, 2012, to increase tobacco taxes for the tenth time in 18 years, from 55% of the factory price in 1992 to 87% in 2012. Tax increases still are not higher than the inflation rate, though, and the current excise and tax ad valorem rate only accounts for 70% of the retail price of cigarettes.

The most significant legislative changes that have occurred in Thailand since

FCTC ratification are in respect to packaging and labeling. In March 2005, Thailand required all tobacco packages to include one of six specific rotating pictorial health warnings, a recommendation contained in the FCTC. Over the following eight years, additional changes were made to the labeling and packaging law. In March 2006, the size of the warnings was increased from the minimum FCTC requirement of 30% of the front and back to the FCTC-recommended size of 50%. In March 2007, the terms "light" and "mild" were banned in accordance with FCTC recommendations, and additional misleading terms were banned in December 2011. Based on this work, at the fourteenth World Conference on Tobacco or Health in 2009, the first Bloomberg Award for Tobacco Control was given to Dr. Prakit Vathisathokit for effectively implementing pictorial health warnings on tobacco products in his role as executive secretary of ASH Thailand. But Thailand was still not done with warning labels.

The size of the warnings was once again increased to 55% of the front and back in March 2010, and to 60% in July 2011. As of January 2012, rotating messages indicating toxic substances are required to appear on the packages as well. Finally, in March 2013, Thailand announced that it would increase the size of its warnings to cover 85% of the front and back of packages—making it the global leader in warning size. In Australia, the previous global leader, warnings cover 75% of the front and 90% of the back of cigarette packs (82.5% on average). The updated Thai package warnings depict the negative effects of smoking, and the top portion of cigarette packages are required to display tobacco cessation information, including a quitline number.

The new warnings were supposed to go into effect in October 2013, but in August 2013, a Thai court granted tobacco companies a temporary stay after they argued that the government acted beyond its powers in increasing the size of the warnings. The government is appealing that decision, but the process is sure to be long and signals yet another battle between the transnational tobacco industry and the Thai government. There is fear that the cases will also be brought to trade bodies in the future. Philip Morris is expected to fight especially hard against Thailand's health warning law (eventually using international trade courts) given the size of the Thai tobacco market.

Although the Thai government has sought to fulfill its FCTC obligations, there are many other areas of FCTC-related legislation that are missing in Thailand. Areas of ongoing debate include legislation around crop diversification or subsidies. Work on viable alternative crops has begun recently after Thailand partnered with the COP working group on economically sustainable alternatives to tobacco cultivation. Other measures such as those pertaining to filing lawsuits for compensation from tobacco harm and protection of the environment from tobacco cultivation are still lacking. An additional challenge in Thailand is the popularity of roll-your-own (RYO) cigarettes. Current Thai legislation focuses on factory-made cigarettes. The excise tax on RYO cigarettes (0.1%) is much lower than that on factory-made ones (85%), and only one of the two pictorial health warnings labels in black and white are required to be displayed on RYO cigarette packaging.

Tobacco Industry Interference

Transnational tobacco companies have remained focused on Thailand since their initial disputes in the late 1980s. Thailand is one of four primary growth markets in Asia; the other three are Indonesia, the Philippines, and Vietnam. The companies have used their considerable financial resources to build up political leverage over time. Given their confrontational relationship with the transnational tobacco companies, Thai advocates have been developing systems for identifying and counteracting transnational tobacco company interference for decades.

There have been numerous cases of tobacco industry activity in Thailand since ratification of the FCTC. One particularity blatant event occurred in 2009 when *Tobacco Reporter*, a US-based magazine, held its annual TABINFO conference in Bangkok, billing it as "the biggest tobacco exhibition in Asia." In advertising for the conference, the trade publication highlighted the size of the Southeast Asian market, writing, "It is also one of the most promising markets in terms of value."[62] The choice of Bangkok for the conference was seen as a direct affront by the tobacco industry to the Thai government's tough actions on tobacco control, and Thai advocates were able to successfully mobilize opposition. Prime Minister Abhisit Vejjajiva, who has said he was unaware of the conference until two weeks before it started, ordered government and tourism agencies not to do anything to promote or support it after activists presented him with a petition that contained more than 82,000 signatures opposing the conference. After opposition to the conference gained momentum, Thailand's state-run tobacco monopoly withdrew its exhibitions and sponsorship of a buffet breakfast for industry representatives just days before the conference began. More than 600 protestors invaded the convention center before being forced to leave by security guards, and the conference organizers refused to meet with the protestors and locked the meeting room doors to members of the media.

The key goal of the international tobacco companies has been a strategy of localization: becoming Thai rather than foreign.[63] Thai tobacco control advocates

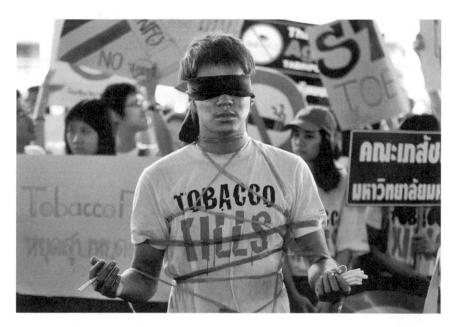

Figure 11. A Thai student takes part in a protest against the tobacco exposition TABINFO Asia, which was held in Bangkok, Thailand, in November 2009. Several hundred students took part in the protest during the three-day exposition. Associated Press Photo / Apichart Weerawong

have for years successfully branded the international tobacco companies as foreign imperialists. Consequently, the more effectively the international tobacco companies can localize, the more effectively they can undermine the Thai tobacco control messages of the past. The companies have attempted to weaken the strong opposition to the industry from the media and promote their local message by creating their own network of sympathetic reporters and columnists. The companies have nurtured these relationships by giving journalists special treatment such as overseas trips.[64] They have also supported the Thai Tobacco Growers, Curers, and Dealers Association (TTA), which has lobbied the Thai government not to agree with FCTC articles 9–10 in relation to the regulation of the content of tobacco products and disclosures, arguing that such regulation would substantially reduce demand for their crops, resulting in farmers losing their jobs.

Thai tobacco control advocates have turned to the FCTC to counteract the growing influence of the transnational companies. In 2004, advocates achieved a new cabinet directive barring tobacco companies from making financial or material contributions to government officials or engaging in political activities. The guidelines of article 5.3 (tobacco industry interference), adopted at the third COP in Durban, South Africa in November 2008, provided additional support of this directive. Following COP3, Ritthiphakdee told the press, "Fortunately we are now having the guidelines of WHO FCTC article 5.3 on protection of public health policies from tobacco industry interference, which asked the government of each party to have clear policy of not allowing the tobacco's industry's interference."[65]

Unfortunately, the FCTC has not protected Thailand from industry-driven litigation, and trade litigation has continued to plague Thai tobacco control during the past decade. In September 2008, the Philippines filed a case with the World Trade Organization that challenged Thailand for "biased, partial, and unreasonable" administration of its tobacco tax measures, which give an advantage to the TTM, the main competitor of Filipino cigarettes in the Thai cigarette market. The Philippines claimed that Thailand was overvaluing imported cigarettes at customs, resulting in tariffs and taxes being charged at higher rates than were due. The Philippines also claimed that the tax system was administered in a discriminatory manner, partly because the methodologies used for calculating taxes favored domestic producers. The WTO panel agreed that the tax system was administered in a discriminatory manner. Thailand appealed that decision, but the WTO's appellate body upheld the panel's report.

Civil Society

The line between government official and civil society activist has never been entirely clear in Thailand. Like in many low- and middle-income countries, highly successful professionals often take on multiple roles, such as clinician, politician, and advocate. For the first decade of tobacco control in Thailand, a committed group of less than a dozen such tobacco control advocates managed to mobilize social support for tobacco control, gather evidence, counter the transnational tobacco companies, and push for ever-stronger legislation and enforcement. With the support of foreign funding agencies, small-scale research and capacity building grew in the early 2000s. Thai researchers increasingly took part in large multi-country research protocols and extended their research into the policy-making arena.[66] Since 2001, some of the individual power of agency that defined tobacco control in Thailand for so long has been translated into structural power through ThaiHealth. ThaiHealth now provides domestic support for locally relevant research and implementation of evidence-based programs.

ThaiHealth has provided the foundation on which to build a much larger support base for tobacco control. In 2005, ThaiHealth supported the formation of Thai Health Professionals Against Tobacco (THPAT) and the Teachers Against Tobacco Network (TATN). These associations have achieved greater involvement of health professionals and teachers in tobacco control, as demonstrated by their increased participation in regional and international conferences. For example, 95 Thais participated in the 2010 Asia Pacific Conference on Tobacco or Health (APACT) in Sydney—the largest contingent from outside of Australia. The decades of civil society engagement in tobacco control, including the multiple confrontations with the tobacco industry, have resulted in widespread awareness and support for tobacco control among the general public.

The establishment of ThaiHealth has also had a positive impact on domestic tobacco control research. A study of Thai tobacco control research ten years before (1990–2000) and after (2001–2011) the creation of ThaiHealth found a fivefold increase in both the number of publications (74 vs. 376) and the number of Thai-based first authors.[67] Multiple Thai universities, including Mahidol and Thammasat, have tobacco control researchers that receive support from domestic and international funders. The ThaiHealth model, with tobacco control as the core of health promotion, is now being promoted across the Southeast Asia region and globally as a way for low- and middle-income countries to build capacity and sustain funding in chronic disease prevention and care.[68]

In addition to these domestic organizations, SEATCA continues to provide a forum for advocacy in Thailand and throughout the region. Ritthiphakdee represents one of very few Asians to have worked full time on tobacco control for more than 20 years. As she has widened her field of activities as SEATCA's director, her experience and leadership have become an invaluable resource for the region and for the world. She has received ongoing global recognition for her work, including the Luther Terry Award from the American Cancer Society in 2006 and an honorable mention by the editors of the Asian editions of *Reader's Digest* in the Asian of the Year 2010 Awards.

Ritthiphakdee's leadership of SEATCA has most recently focused on challenging the placement of tobacco in international trade agreements, specifically supporting Malaysia's proposal to exclude tobacco from the Trans-Pacific Partnership (TPP) trade agreement. After the United States failed to put forward the proposal as expected (described in Chapter 4), members of the Southeast Asian tobacco control community, including Ritthiphakdee, went into action drafting a proposal and gaining support from the Malaysian government for its submission to the negotiations. In defending the Malaysian proposal, Ritthiphakdee pointed to the tobacco industry's use of trade-related arguments to undermine and derail the Thai government's tobacco control measures.[69]

Thailand's compliance with the FCTC is the result of more than two decades of sustained effort. The treaty did not initiate tobacco control efforts in Thailand, but it has provided a credible foundation for ongoing efforts to strengthen existing regulations, build greater infrastructure, and counter industry influence. Thailand is a prime example of a middle-income country that drove the successful completion of the FCTC process, and it illustrates how advocates can continue to use the instrument to impact domestic policy. Although much has been achieved, new challenges continue to arise, including stalled decreases in consumption and new industry strategies to undermine effective control policies.

Gone are the days when Thai advocates were clueless as to the threats of transnational companies or were in need of technical handholding from international experts. Today, Thai tobacco control professionals are global experts in their own right, actively assisting advocates in other high-, middle-, and low-income countries in their efforts to counter the tobacco epidemic. They not only have the expertise, but they have secured the domestic resources required for a sustained program that promises to save millions of lives in Thailand and throughout the Southeast Asian region.

But Thai tobacco control advocates have not had it easy. They have faced intense industry opposition, legislative corruption, and an ongoing lack of commitment from many policymakers. Their astonishing success in this context over the past two decades should provide inspiration to those in the midst of pushing for tobacco control in countries where many politicians still value and promote the tobacco industry. The experience of Thai tobacco control advocates illustrates how a low- or middle-income country can move from adapting international evidence and best practices to unique domestic contexts, to building the political commitment needed to formally institutionalize and sustainably fund tobacco control in a country. The Thai story also demonstrates the lengths it takes, personal and institutional, to ensure that sound, evidence-based legislation is passed and implemented in a highly politicized world. Thailand's ongoing struggles with transnational tobacco companies, moreover, show the depth of technical and financial commitment it takes to sustain a national program for decades.

CHAPTER SIX

The FCTC in Uruguay

Igniting a Global Leader

At the turn of the twenty-first century, Uruguay was among the most tobacco-friendly countries in Latin America. Tobacco control policies were limited and ineffective, and tobacco prevalence and consumption, though similar to that of its larger neighbor Argentina, was much higher than in most other Latin American countries. At the time of the Framework Convention on Tobacco Control negotiations, Uruguay was perhaps best known in tobacco control circles for the international outrage it caused in 2002 when the Uruguayan World Cup soccer team was officially sponsored by the Nevada brand of cigarettes.[1] The sponsorship was especially newsworthy at the time because the opening of the World Cup coincided with the launch of a major international campaign led by the Tobacco Free Initiative entitled "Tobacco Free Sports—Play It Clean."[2] The campaign focused specifically on the need to reject tobacco sponsorship of athletic teams and sporting events, and Uruguay's actions were seen as a direct challenge to TFI's efforts.[3]

Remarkably, within a decade Uruguay would transform from a global tobacco control dissenter into the first country in the world to implement every one of the FCTC obligations and nearly all recommendations. As a newly crowned global tobacco control innovator, Uruguay would also become a key test case in resisting tobacco industry efforts to block domestic tobacco control regulations using international trade agreements.

Uruguay did not make its tobacco control transformation in isolation. Uruguayan tobacco control advocates and policymakers received extensive technical, financial, and moral support from the international tobacco control community. Much of this support was directly linked to initiatives supporting the ratification and implementation of the FCTC. Consequently, Uruguay serves as a testament to the impact that international political processes can have on domestic policy. In Uruguay, strong executive leadership and close collaboration among a committed Ministry of Health (MOH) and dedicated non-governmental advocates with strong external funding support enhanced the treaty's impact.

Pre-FCTC Tobacco Control in Uruguay

Before 2000 and the start of the FCTC process, tobacco and tobacco control received very little attention in Uruguay. Only 0.3% of the country's population of 3.3 million was employed by the tobacco industry, and tobacco contributed roughly 0.4% of gross domestic product.[4] The domestic tobacco company Monte Paz controlled more than 70% of the domestic market, whereas Philip Morris controlled approximately 20%, having made its original investment in Uruguay in 1979 by acquiring Abal Hermanos SA. The only other transnational tobacco company present in the country was British American Tobacco, which controlled an estimated 1% of the market.[5]

Tobacco products in Uruguay had always been very inexpensive. In the late 1990s, the cheapest cigarette in the country (Montana cigarettes, produced by BAT) cost approximately $1 for a pack of 20 cigarettes, whereas a pack of 20 Nevada cigarettes (Monte Paz's most popular brand) cost just slightly more than $1. Packs of international brands such as Marlboro cost less than $2.[6]

Regardless of its limited contribution to the domestic economy, the tobacco lobby managed to systematically block all tobacco control bills proposed in the Uruguayan parliament for more than 25 years. The few regulations in place came from executive decrees, and even they were not enforced. In 1996, for example, a decree was passed implementing partial restrictions on smoking in public places, but it was never enforced and smoking remained heavy in public places.

In addition to the lack of regulations, Uruguay also lacked the scientific evidence base supporting tobacco control, including any form of national surveillance system for tobacco consumption and related social, economic, and health indicators. Based on small surveys, the men's smoking prevalence rate was estimated at approximately 38%, whereas the women's rate was 27%.[7] The Global Youth Tobacco Survey, conducted for the first time in Uruguay in 2001, found that boys' and girls' rates of smoking were equal at approximately 23%.[8] Given the lack of tobacco control regulations, the most important determinant of tobacco sales was household income, with rises in household income linked to higher tobacco sales and vice versa.[9] In the late 1990s, Uruguay faced significant decreases in household income, and cigarette sales decreased accordingly.

Until the end of the twentieth century, support for tobacco control was primarily limited to a small handful of prominent doctors in Uruguay who advocated on the sidelines for smoking cessation and greater tobacco regulation. The

Commission to Fight Cancer in Uruguay, for example, had promoted smoking restrictions in public places since the late 1980s.[10,11]

The FCTC Process in Uruguay

The Uruguayan government was very slow to engage in the FCTC process. Although technical delegates, including representatives from the MOH, Cancer Honorary Commission, Hospital de Clínicas, and at one point a representative of the National Drug Commission, were sent to the negotiations in Geneva, they lacked a specific negotiating mandate from the government. Uruguay's active participation in the final negotiating session in 2003 was the result of an effort started years before by members of civil society committed to achieving a strong FCTC.

One key individual in this effort was Dr. Eduardo Bianco. In 1999, as a national leader in the growing smoking cessation movement, Dr. Bianco attended the Second Ibero-American Congress in Las Palmas, Gran Canaria, Spain. There Dr. Bianco met some of the senior global tobacco control leaders who enlightened him to the tactics of the transnational tobacco companies and introduced him to the FCTC. After this conference, Dr. Bianco returned to Uruguay committed to convincing one of the medical associations of which he was a member to engage in the FCTC process. After failing to convince the Uruguayan Cardiology Society in 1999, he succeeded with Sindicato Médico del Uruguay (SMU) in 2000.

In that same year, SMU began attending, quite by accident, periodic meetings between the MOH and local Pan American Health Organization (PAHO) staff. Through these meetings, SMU began informing the MOH and PAHO staff about the FCTC process and the need for Uruguay to participate more actively. SMU also began inviting other NGOs supportive of tobacco control to these meetings, including the highly influential Inland Medical Federation and the Montevideo Municipality. Together, these groups quickly succeeded in convincing the Health Services Office of the Ministry of Public Health to request formation of the National Alliance for Tobacco Control (henceforth referred to as the Alliance) to support government efforts to control tobacco.[12]

The establishment of the Alliance provided a major boost to Uruguay's tobacco control movement. Its mission was to enhance domestic tobacco control capacity and to eventually create a national tobacco control policy that would help lower the prevalence of smoking and protect the population from involuntary exposure to secondhand smoke. In total, the Alliance included 14 national organizations representing governmental, quasi-governmental, private, and grassroots organizations, and it was endorsed by PAHO. The Alliance's strength derived from the broad spectrum of member organizations, including public institutions responsible for formulating national health and drug policies, as well as important medical institutions (the National Medical School, the Medical Union, and the Inland Medical Federation).[13]

Financial support for the Alliance initially came from its members, but it eventually succeeded in obtaining support from international organizations and foundations, including the American Cancer Society (ACS), the American Heart Association, the Canadian Heart Foundation, the InterAmerican Heart Foundation (IAHF), and PAHO. Later on, support also came from the Framework Convention Alliance (FCA), the Canadian International Development Research Center (IDRC), and the Campaign for Tobacco-Free Kids.

A fundamental objective of the Alliance from its inception was to raise awareness about the FCTC and advocate for Uruguay's participation.[14] In 2001, SMU held the first National Tobacco Control Meeting focused on the FCTC. Members of the Alliance participated in regional FCTC negotiations before Intergovernmental Negotiating Body 2 (INB2) and at the global level beginning at INB3 as members of NGOs. In 2002, Dr. Bianco became the director of the Tobacco Control Program at IAHF and the Latin American coordinator of the FCA.

The experiences, connections, and materials gained from this international work were shared throughout the Alliance and helped Uruguayan advocates organize themselves domestically and prepare the groundwork for the future. Although the government did not immediately become active in the FCTC, the Alliance continued to advocate for the MOH to adopt a position in support of a strong FCTC and encouraged it to work with other ministries, such as the Ministry of Education and Culture and the Ministry of Economy and Finance, in defining Uruguay's positions on specific articles in the draft text. Finally, in 2003, as a consequence of the Alliance's pressure and increasing activity in the MOH on tobacco control issues, Uruguay sent a formal delegation to the final negotiating session in Geneva with a clear mandate to support a strong FCTC.

Obviously, Uruguay's participation in the FCTC negotiations was much too little and too late to have any real influence on the treaty text. However, the country's last-minute participation in the FCTC process initiated cross-sectoral collaboration and increased press coverage and domestic debate regarding tobacco control. It also reflected a domestic change on tobacco control during the previous three years that was initially supported by the PAHO Smoke-Free Americas

Initiative. In 2000, civil society members were invited by PAHO to attend a regional meeting in Rio de Janeiro, Brazil, where the FCTC process was presented and advocates were encouraged to engage. In 2001, members of the Alliance were again invited to participate in a workshop convened by PAHO in Foz do Iguaçu, Brazil, as part of its Smoke-Free Americas Initiative. The workshop focused on developing national action plans to promote smoke-free environments. Based on this meeting, the Alliance developed a project calling for the designation of areas where smoking was prohibited in municipal government offices in Montevideo, as well as in Hospital de Clínicas, a hospital affiliated with the Universidad de la República. This project resulted in some of the first press coverage of smoke-free environments in Uruguay.[15]

Also as part of the PAHO Smoke-Free Americas Initiative, the Alliance participated in a multi-country research study measuring levels of nicotine in the air in public places, such as hospitals, offices, high schools, airports, bars, and restaurants. The goal of the study was to collect evidence of secondhand smoke exposure in capital cities to support smoking bans throughout the region. The results of the study in Uruguay revealed high levels of tobacco smoke in all places studied, including in schools and healthcare facilities.[16] Comparatively speaking, Uruguay and Argentina shared the dubious distinction of having the highest levels of tobacco smoke pollution in South America. The results of the study generated a great deal of press and served as the foundation of a 2004 presidential decree banning smoking in all healthcare facilities in the country.[17]

In 2003, PAHO invited MOH Director General, Dr. Diego Estol, and members of the Alliance to a Smoke-Free Americas Initiative workshop held in Jamaica. The workshop was officially for Caribbean countries, but Uruguay was invited as an observer to assess if such workshops would be applicable in Latin America. The involvement of both the MOH leadership and the Alliance members at the workshop led to enhanced collaboration between the two organizations and a growing commitment to work together on smoke-free policies in Uruguay. Subsequently, a second PAHO Smoke-Free Americas Initiative workshop, the first in Latin America, was held in Uruguay in 2003. This workshop provided the government and other Alliance members the opportunity to advocate for the creation of smoke-free environments among its organizational members, invited policymakers, and the press.[18]

Building on the momentum of the workshop, PAHO granted the Alliance $15,000 to work on smoke-free places in the country. This funding supported collaborative work between Dr. Estol at the MOH and the Alliance on Project Smoke-Free Uruguay.[19] The project aimed to make all health and educational

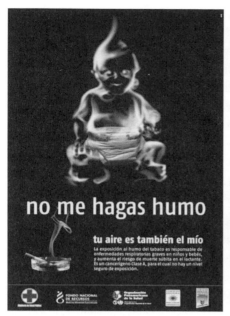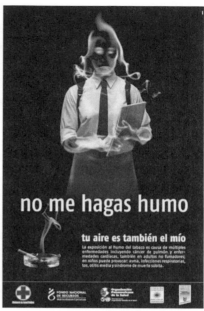

Figure 12. "Don't Make Me Smoke" campaign image. Agencia Perfil, commissioned by the World Health Organization, Prevention of Non-communicable Diseases

facilities and public offices 100% smoke free in a period of 24 months.[20] As part of the project, a mass media campaign entitled "Don't make me smoke . . . we breathe the same air" was launched. The campaign consisted of posters with information and graphic images on the harms of exposure to secondhand smoke. The campaign also included three radio jingles based on famous advertising spots, one of which won the 2005 award for radio spots from the Uruguayan Chamber of Advertisers' Global Bell Competition.[21] Informational pamphlets and smoke-free environment stickers were also distributed to businesses and offices throughout the country. Through Project Smoke-Free Uruguay, the Alliance grew into a recognized, vocal, and well-connected entity that was closely associated with the Uruguayan government.

FCTC Ratification and Entry into Force

Uruguay signed the FCTC in June 2003, less than a month after the World Health Assembly adopted it. However, ratification of the FCTC required a parliamentary vote; thus, the Alliance had to build broad support among policymakers largely unfamiliar with tobacco control. Moreover, unlike many other countries in which FCTC-compatible tobacco legislation was already in place, the Alliance had to convince Uruguayan policymakers to commit to an agreement that implied wide and sweeping policy shifts in the domestic tobacco control environment. The upcoming national elections in October 2004 put additional pressure on tobacco control advocates to work quickly and have the treaty ratified before a new government took office.

During the following year, the Alliance received international funding from organizations to support their efforts to ratify the FCTC. With this support, they undertook an extensive study of how ratification could best be achieved while avoiding bureaucratic red tape, identified strong new allies to accelerate ratification, and built public awareness in support of the FCTC. SMU called on the National Resources Fund (FNR) to support their efforts, which was a well-respected and well-funded organization dedicated to expanding access in Uruguay to expensive, high-quality medical interventions such as cardiac surgery and angioplasties. FNR agreed to support tobacco control and wrote letters and contacted parliamentarians requesting rapid FCTC ratification. Alliance members held meetings with the health commissions of each house of parliament, and they held interviews with representatives and senators from the four political parties in the country. They worked tirelessly with lawmakers interested in the issue.[22] Leadership by Dr. Estol at the MOH was critical to maintaining momentum. Dr. Tabaré Vázquez (then Montevideo City mayor and leader of his political party) was key in convincing his political party, Frente Amplio, to vote unanimously in favor of ratification.

Domestic press coverage also helped shift opinions among the general population and policymakers. Much of this press coverage was supported by international grants, including those from the ACS and IAHF, which supported journalism training workshops and competitions. These activities provided the opportunity to engage many significant Uruguayan journalists in tobacco control, including Carlos Maggi, Juan Carlos Paullier, Leonardo Haberkorn, and others. These individuals continued to support tobacco control long after the trainings and competitions ended.

In July 2004, the Uruguayan parliament approved ratification of the FCTC, and Uruguay officially ratified the treaty on September 9, 2004, just one month before national elections.[23] Uruguay was the third Latin American country to ratify, following Mexico and Panama, and the ratification represented a major achievement on the part of the Alliance. Global recognition came to the Alliance in 2005 when it received WHO's World No Tobacco Day Award for securing ratification of the FCTC in Uruguay.[24]

Since ratification, Uruguay has been an active participant in the Conference of Parties, even hosting the fourth COP session in Punta del Este. Members of the Uruguayan delegation have taken leadership roles, including the election of Ambassador Ricardo Varela as COP President at COP4. Uruguay has been a key ally to those seeking strong implementation guidelines, and it is one of the "countries are doing it" examples referred to by Brazilian activist Paula Jones.[25]

Post-FCTC Tobacco Control in Uruguay

Following the ratification of the FCTC and its entry into force in February 2005, the extensive power of the Uruguayan executive branch was used to enact policies through decrees, which are not subject to parliamentary approval, to quickly bring Uruguay in line with its FCTC obligations. Before FCTC ratification, only a few executive decrees concerning tobacco control had ever been issued. In 2003, for example, a decree was passed raising cigarette taxes from 66.5% to 68.7%,[26] but this did not represent a significant rise in tax or price of cigarettes. In 2003, the text of health warning labels was also changed, although the overall tenor remained close to what it had been in the past: "Smoking may lead to cancer, heart disease, and lung disease. Smoking during pregnancy is harmful to your baby."[27] In 2004, a decree was issued that banned smoking in healthcare facilities—a direct outcome of Project Smoke-Free Uruguay.[28] These decrees were limited in scope and did little to change the existing status quo in Uruguay tobacco control policy.

After ratification, decrees were issued at a dizzying pace and covered tobacco taxes, public smoking, warning labels, and tobacco product packaging. Two key events drove the active engagement of the executive branch during this period. The first was the establishment in late 2004 of the Honorary MOH Tobacco Control Advisory Commission (MOH Committee). During the final days of the FCTC negotiations and ratification process, civil society members built strong personal relationships with staff of the MOH, especially with Dr. Estol. To assure greater civil society participation and ongoing momentum in tobacco control in the next government, Dr. Estol proposed to Minister of Health Dr. Conrado Bonilla that they create an honorary committee including NGOs, MOH staff, and other representatives.

The influence of the MOH Committee was instantaneous. At its first meeting in early January 2005, members of civil society asked a MOH legal advisor how they could get health warning labels to cover 50% of the front and back of tobacco packaging. The advisor informed them that although the MOH could not change the text of the warnings, they could define the size immediately. On January 25, 2005, decree 36/005 was issued requiring health warning labels to cover 50% of both principal display areas (front and back) of cigarette packages.[29] The decree entered into force on July 27, 2005.

The second event to drive the participation of the executive branch in tobacco control policy was the election of President Tabaré Vázquez, who was an oncologist by training, familiar with the deadly consequences of tobacco use, and personally committed to tobacco control. President Vázquez had already been influential in achieving ratification of the FCTC. After taking office in March 2005, he did not hesitate to make tobacco control a national priority. Using their direct access to the president, the MOH Committee began making requests that would alter the landscape of tobacco control in Uruguay and around the world.

The first request was for President Vázquez to make a tobacco control policy speech on May 31, 2005, his first World No Tobacco Day in office. In this speech, he laid out a number of groundbreaking tobacco control actions, including the official formation of the MOH Tobacco Control Program. He also announced decree 171/05, which banned misleading terms such as *light, ultra light,* and *mild* on cigarette packages.[30,31] The decree specifically gave the Ministry of Health the right to determine what would be allowed on cigarette packages, including warning label content, and made it responsible for imposing fines on violators.

Subsequently, with the full support of the president, the MOH announced that it would require warnings on cigarette packs to include rotating pictograms on each side.[32] This requirement was an enormous leap from the requirement taken only two years before to include the word "may" on packages in relation to smoking as a cause of cancer. Tobacco companies were given six months to comply, and by April 1, 2006, all cigarette packages sold legally in Uruguay had one of eight graphic health warning labels on both primary display areas: one concerning the harms of secondhand smoke, and the other concerning the consequences of active smoking.

Also as part of his 2005 World No Tobacco Day speech, President Vázquez issued a decree banning direct incentives such as giveaways and tobacco advertisement and promotions relating to sports events, as well as limiting the hours during which cigarette commercials could be aired on television.[33] This decree concerning restrictions on tobacco advertising, promotion, and sponsorship was weak compared to other decrees issued by President Vázquez at the time. The tobacco industry continued to advertise on television after 10 PM and in magazines, and it continued to hold promotional activities unrelated to sports. One final act of President Vázquez's speech was decree 146/005, which raised taxes from 68.7% to 70% on cigarettes, 40% to 41% on cigars, and 27% to 28% on hand-rolled tobacco.[34] Although not substantial tax hikes, these were the first of many increases over the next five years that would culminate in a significant rise in price.

Before the 2005 speech, the MOH Committee asked the president to decree a 100% indoor smoking ban in the country. At the same time, other advisors argued that it was too radical a step so early in his term. During the speech, President Vázquez announced his intention to move toward a 100% smoke free law incrementally, starting with a limited ban that had exceptions for designated smoking rooms. The committee members accepted his incremental approach initially, but did not relent and continued to ask him to exert his leadership on the issue of smoke-free public places.

A key moment for President Vázquez to exhibit this leadership came in August 2005, when the FCA requested that he speak at a regional workshop, Tobacco Control Development for Legislators in Buenos Aires, Argentina. Just before the workshop, a distinguished delegation of international tobacco control experts visited the president and advocated that he call for 100% smoke-free environments during his speech. Consequently, on August 17, 2005, President Vázquez lectured on the importance of tobacco control policy development, including 100% smoke-free air policies, in Buenos Aires, and a few weeks later on September 5, 2005, he released another decree banning smoking in all indoor workplaces, on public transport, and in public places.[35,36] On March 1, 2006, the decree entered into force and Uruguay became the first country in the Americas—and the third in the world—to be totally smoke free.

During the course of one year, Uruguay went from almost no tobacco control policies to complying with the FCTC recommendations in regard to the packaging and labeling of tobacco products and public smoking bans. These abrupt changes were accomplished without one formal vote on tobacco control policy by the Uruguayan parliament. President Vázquez was awarded the WHO World No Tobacco Day Award in 2006 for his leadership in tobacco control.[37]

Enforcement and Public Campaigns

Although countries may have tobacco control policies in place, many fail to implement and enforce those policies. Policy compliance can be especially challenging in low- and middle-income countries that lack capacity for enforcement and for executing mass public education campaigns. The speed at which the new decrees were issued in Uruguay posed a significant challenge to effective enforcement, leaving little time to prepare the population for the new laws. The MOH Tobacco Control Program established by President Vázquez in May 2005 was responsible for tobacco control policy, programming, monitoring, and enforcement. The majority of the government's attention to enforcement focused on the public smoking ban. Packaging and labeling requirements on legal tobacco products do not require much enforcement because they are standardized at the point of manufacturing and few companies are in the Uruguayan tobacco market.

In regard to the smoking ban in public places, the decree included sanctions for violations by owners or managers that permitted smoking. The sanctions were $1,200 for first offense, $2,400 for second offense, and up to a three-day closure for a third offense.[38] In relation to the standard of living in Uruguay, these fines represented a significant deterrent. The day that the decree went into force, the Ministry of Public Health deployed teams of inspectors and entered into agreements with other public institutions and municipal government offices throughout the country to enforce the decree. Through the MOH Committee, NGOs also played key roles in monitoring the enforcement of policies and programs, including the public smoking ban. Although differences occasionally arise, the various stakeholders in the MOH committee share the same objectives and rely on each other to achieve their goals. Strong interpersonal relationships built through the years and fluent communication between the committee and other members of civil society facilitate their coordinated efforts. In regard to the national smoking ban, civil society enforcement is coordinated through the Red por un Uruguay Libre de Tabaco (RULTA) or Smokefree Uruguay Network, originally established in 2003 by SMU and the Passive Smokers Association.[39]

Perhaps surprisingly given the overnight nature of the smoking ban, public compliance with the decree was high from the start. Only two restaurant owners aggressively challenged the ban in the media, insisting that they would not obey the ban.[40] The Ministry of Health immediately fined both owners. The high level of compliance was reflected in the low number of sanctions that were issued by the Ministry of Health after the ban was put in place. After one year, the Ministry of Health had carried out 4,000 inspections and only levied 17 fines.[41]

Compliance with the ban can largely be credited to the massive public education campaigns carried out quickly by the government and civil society partners in the lead up to its entry into force. The Smokefree Uruguay Network, for example, implemented three mass media campaigns in conjunction with the ban. The first, "No me hagas humo" ("Don't make me smoke") aimed at increasing awareness of the dangers of secondhand smoke and rationale for the smoking ban. The second campaign was meant to prepare the public to accept the decree. It was entitled "One Million Thanks," referring to the country's one million smokers. The campaign was launched by President Vázquez himself via videoconference to the whole country,[42] and it included gathering one million signatures to thank those who refrained from smoking in public places. Signatures were collected through leaflets, free phone calls, and a campaign website. In total, more than one million signatures (1,112,643) were collected.[43]

The third campaign was called "Smokefree Uruguay" and was aimed at building popular support for smoke-free places. The campaign focused on the positive aspects of smoke-free places and launched a national logo for a smoke-free environment. The logo identified smoke-free places and standardized the transition to smoke-free environments nationwide. The "Smokefree Uruguay" campaign also included an informational brochure, a television spot, radio spots, and posters. It unfolded during the weeks leading up to the implementation of the smoking ban to help ensure future compliance with the measure.[44]

Another key civil society partner during implementation of the ban was FNR, who was challenged by SMU and launched a smoking cessation program entitled "Quit Smoking Before Life Quits You" in tandem with Project Smoke-free Uruguay.[45] The campaign portrayed smoking as an addiction that is difficult to overcome, provided information about the harm caused by smoking, and offered treatment for free at its facilities. Initially, FNR provided cessation services itself; however, in light of the growing demand, fund officials quickly realized the need to create technical resources capable of providing ongoing smoking cessation services. Accordingly, the FNR trained healthcare professionals (physicians, psychologists, nurses, social workers, dentists, and others) in tobacco dependence treatment and developed agreements with health organizations and institutions, public and private, throughout the country to provide patients with free pharmacological support for tobacco dependence. This program became the foundation of the National Smoking Cessation Program. The trainings also included information about the FCTC. Between 2004 and 2007, FNR delivered training, nicotine replacement therapy, and bupropion for free to more than 100 programs in the country.[46] Dr. Eduardo Bianco was promoted (with SMU) and then appointed to lead the FNR's tobacco dependence treatment strategy.

Before the FNR's involvement in smoking cessation, the Honorary Commission to Fight Cancer offered limited cessation services at the Hospital de Clínicas in Montevideo, and only a few other governmental and private sector service providers offered treatment.[47] The FNR's campaign markedly increased the availability of smoking cessation services nationwide, with many of these services provided free of charge regardless of the individual patient's health coverage.[48] The FNR's focus on treatment was considered critical in the future success of Uruguay's public smoking ban because it promoted smokers' efforts to beat their addiction and made the measures less difficult for smokers, who felt that their needs were being considered.

In November 2006, six months after the implementation of the smoking ban, the Ministry of Public Health, in collaboration with PAHO, conducted a public survey to evaluate the effect of the smoking ban on the population. The survey found that a strong majority (92%) of Uruguayans surveyed agreed that tobacco smoke is hazardous or very hazardous to health, and 94% of respondents agreed that employees had the right to work in an environment free of tobacco smoke. The government survey also found that 94% of the respondents were aware of the decree banning smoking, and an overall 80% (86% of non-smokers, 90% of ex-smokers, and 63% of smokers) of respondents said that they agreed with the decree. The survey results testify to the concerted efforts made by the Vázquez government and civil society partners to publicize the measure and its implementation.

Legislation and National Policy

Although the executive decrees were instrumental in kick-starting Uruguayan tobacco control, they have a lower legal standing than laws and can be repealed easily by subsequent administrations. Laws, alternatively, are far more difficult to amend or repeal. For this reason, tobacco control advocates in Uruguay worked hard to have the contents of the Vázquez government's decrees incorporated into law before he left office. Additionally, the dramatic evolution of tobacco control in Uruguay had not gone unnoticed by the domestic or transnational tobacco industry.

Despite their relatively weak presence in the Uruguayan tobacco market, the transnational tobacco industry had been active for years with policymakers. Although documentary evidence is lacking on expenditures by the transnational tobacco industry on advertising, promotion, or sponsorship in Uruguay, there were clear attempts by the industry to challenge the executive decrees and block the passage of comprehensive tobacco control legislation. When the new health warning label decree was passed, for example, the tobacco industry issued a press release shortly before the regulation went into force characterizing some of the pictograms as "offensive" and "denigrating."[49] With regard to the smoking ban, the industry pushed the idea of freedom of choice, emphasizing that every unnecessary prohibition was an erosion of freedom.

After the smoking ban went into effect, the industry continued to run a media campaign asking for tolerance and inclusion of the smoker in society. Such media campaigns seemed to be targeted at parliamentarians who the industry hoped would roll back the measures contained in the decrees, including reauthorizing smoking areas through formal legislation and preventing any additional advertising restrictions. As was widely reported in the press, the tobacco industry actively lobbied policymakers throughout the debate on a comprehensive law.

One key weakness recognized by tobacco control experts at the time was the lack of domestic evidence and advocacy resources to endorse and support tobacco control policies and counter industry arguments. To address this gap, IDRC encouraged a group of tobacco control advocates and researchers to create an independent research organization to fulfill this role, which it subsequently funded. The Research Center of the Tobacco Epidemic (CIET) was launched in 2006, replacing SMU's former Observatorio Nacional de la Epidemia de Tabaquismo (ONET).

CIET is a multidisciplinary organization that includes healthcare workers, journalists, parliamentarians, economists, lawyers, and others. Its leadership includes Dr. Eduardo Bianco as president and former MOH Director General Dr. Diego Estol as secretary manager. The organization is meant to guide research, capacity building, and advocacy for tobacco control in Uruguay. Specifically, CIET advises the government and civil society on best practices and monitors FCTC implementation in the country. A core project of CIET during its first few years was the implementation of the International Tobacco Control Policy Evaluation Project (ITC) in Uruguay. In Uruguay, ITC has followed a cohort study of approximately 1,400 smokers every two years since 2006.[50] Like elsewhere, the study has proven to be an excellent way to monitor and understand what is happening in the population in regard to tobacco use and control policies and to evaluate the impact of domestic tobacco control policies in line with the FCTC. CIET is formally involved in enforcement activities with the government through the sharing of its evidence.

An experienced and effective lobbying force in its own right, and now with data showing the effective implementation of popular tobacco control laws in force, the Alliance pushed for parliamentary approval of a new tobacco control law that would further institutionalize the executive decrees. Two key individuals helped gain approval for the law: Dr. Miguel Asqueta, a national house representative from 2005 to 2010 and member of the political opposition party, Partido Nacional, and Dr. Gustavo Sóñora, Dr. Asqueta's legal advisor. Both would subsequently take on significant roles in tobacco control organizations at the national and regional levels. Dr. Asqueta would become CIET's vice president and Dr. Sóñora would first become CIET's legal advisor and then regional legal advisor in tobacco control for the International Union Against Lung Disease.

In March 2008, the content of the executive decrees was formally included (and in some cases strengthened) in a groundbreaking national tobacco control law (law 18.256). The law included six strategic points:

(1) 100% smoke-free environments;

(2) supervision of the smoke-free environment regulation;

(3) health warnings with images and captions covering 80% of both principal sides of the package;

(4) a comprehensive advertising ban;

(5) incorporation of diagnosis and treatment of tobacco dependency in public and private health services, including mandatory smoking cessation clinics; and

(6) prohibition of terms, marks, signs, or promotions that create false impressions of certain tobacco products as less harmful than others, including any promotion of these false impressions on cigarette packs.[51]

The law placed Uruguay at the top of the global tobacco control pyramid, with it now having the largest health warnings in the world (at 80%) on cigarette packaging and meeting every one of the gold standards for tobacco control as outlined in the MPOWER measures.[52]

Although the law provided a national tobacco control strategy, it failed to include specific funding for implementation and enforcement. The only organization to directly invest money for tobacco control was the FNR in its support of tobacco dependence treatment. The MOH received some funds from penalties to assist with ongoing smoke-free environment monitoring; however, high compliance had reduced fines as an income source. Efforts to get earmarked taxes for tobacco control programming failed. Most of the research and campaigns continued to be supported by international institutions and organizations, including WHO, PAHO, ACS, the Union for International Cancer Control (UICC), the Campaign for Tobacco-Free Kids, the FCA, the IAHF, the IDRC in Canada, Johns Hopkins University, and others.

In addition to the core legislation, Uruguay also passed progressive tax increases, including a dramatic tax increase that went into place in 2010. Overall,

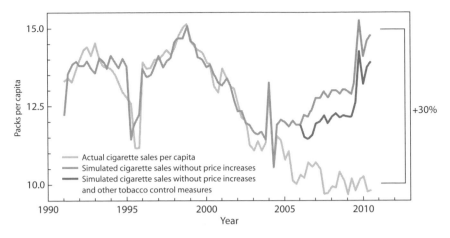

Figure 13. Projected cigarette sales in the absence of price increases and other tobacco control measures in Uruguay, 1991–2010.

between 2005 and 2010 cigarette prices rose from $1.17 to more than $3.00 per pack. There is evidence that the sequential tax increases between 2005 and 2010 have had a positive effect on decreasing tobacco use. Since 2005, household incomes have increased significantly (almost 36% in a few years), and cigarette sales have continued to decrease in spite of rising income. Researchers estimate that if the tax measures had not been implemented, tobacco sales would have been 28% higher.[53]

However, studies show that only 40% of current Uruguayan smokers think about the money they spend on smoking, which suggests that there is still room for future price increases.[54] Additional efforts to raise taxes have been challenged by the belief still pervasive among Uruguayan policymakers that further tax increases will lead to even greater smuggling (a notion promoted by the tobacco industry). According to results from the ITC, approximately 14% of smokers in Uruguay report that their cigarette pack had either no warning label or a nonstandard warning label indicating that they are foreign cigarettes.[55] Tax evasion or illicit cigarette trade is particularly a problem in border communities in Uruguay where smokers can easily cross the border with Paraguay to purchase foreign cigarettes. There is currently no legislation in Uruguay regarding smuggled cigarettes, and there are no enforcement measures to limit the sale of smuggled cigarettes. Accordingly, tobacco activists argue that tobacco smuggling is one of the weakest areas of tobacco control in Uruguay, undermining package and labeling requirements as well as efforts to increase the price of tobacco products through taxation.[56]

Ongoing Industry Opposition

Following the passage of its national tobacco control law, Uruguay became an international flash point between public health advocates and the transnational tobacco industry. In 2010, Philip Morris International (PMI) filed a request for arbitration against Uruguay under the Switzerland-Uruguay bilateral investment treaty. PMI alleged that the provisions of Uruguay's tobacco regulations went beyond reasonable public health regulations. The two measures that formed the basis of PMI's final treaty claim were: (1) Presidential Decree 287/009 (issued June 15, 2009; entered into force December 12, 2009), in which the existing mandate for 50% of the bottom portion of all cigarette packs to contain prescribed health messages was increased to 80%; and (2) Ordinance 514 (issued August 18, 2009; entered into force February 14, 2010), in which existing prohibitions on the use of misleading product names (such as *light* or *mild*) were extended to limit the use of brands to a single line of products.[57]

The most important claim in the PMI suit is related to the single product clause of the law. Indeed, the most valuable asset of the tobacco industry is not plants, equipment, or products, but the branding of its products. The tobacco industry invests greatly in its trademarks because premium brands afford considerably higher profit margins for tobacco producers and importers than generics.[58] Tobacco companies maximize the value of their brands by applying them to an entire family of products. For example, PMI has dozens of variations of its Marlboro brand in different markets worldwide. As regulations banning specific branding such as *light* and *mild* have gone into effect, companies have effectively used color coding to communicate different brand lines. Uruguay's regulation to a single product challenges this worldwide practice of numerous tobacco companies.

The timing of the PMI case is noteworthy because it was filed just as President Vázquez was leaving office. There was great uncertainty at the time about whether the new president, Jose Mujica, would defend the tobacco control efforts of his predecessor. He was a heavy smoker himself and was known as the world's "poorest" president.[59] Mujica publically worried that Uruguay, with a gross domestic product of approximately $44 billion, could not compete against PMI's $108 billion business. When the case was first filed, he called for a negotiated exit, arguing that the country did not have resources for "contract lawyers at $1,500 an hour for several years."[60]

From the beginning of the case, PMI's actions were viewed in Uruguay and around the world as an attempt to bully a small, relatively poor country to weaken its tobacco control regulations and, thus, intimidate other low- and middle-income countries that cannot afford to engage in expensive litigation. Michael Bloomberg and other international tobacco control advocates quickly recognized the potential ripple effects if Uruguay bent to tobacco industry pressure, and they believed it was critically important to defend Uruguay against the tobacco giants. Consequently, Bloomberg offered Uruguay the technical and financial support required to defend the law.[61] Since then, the two sides have fought to set a global precedent for health, trade, and the rights of transnational companies in regard to domestic regulations. The final outcome of the case promises to be years off as it inches through the bureaucratic court procedures and processes.

While the PMI case makes its way slowly through the litigation process, the groundbreaking policies remain in force in Uruguay, and its tobacco control campaign serves as a test case and model for efforts in other low- and middle-income countries. There is growing evidence that Uruguay's comprehensive tobacco control legislation and programs, including its large graphic health warnings, have been associated with substantial, and unprecedented, decreases in tobacco use. Per person consumption of cigarettes in Uruguay decreased by 4.3% per year from 2005 to 2011. Among youth, 30-day prevalence of tobacco use decreased by an estimated 8% per year. Also during 2005–2011, the prevalence of current tobacco use in Uruguay decreased annually by an estimated 3.3% (equivalent to 23% over 6 years).[62] This reduction is more than twice the level of decline seen in neighboring Argentina, which is not party to the FCTC, during the same period. In addition, after Uruguay banned smoking in all enclosed public spaces and workplaces in 2006, air nicotine concentrations and hospital admissions for acute myocardial infarction decreased substantially.

Perhaps in no other country is the impact of international forces on the course of national tobacco control more obvious. From the initial engagement of PAHO through its Smoke-Free Americas Initiative, to the advocacy support from the ACS, IDRC, IAHF, and others, to the financial backing of Michael Bloomberg in the ongoing trade dispute, international organizations and individuals have partnered with local advocates to build national capacity, advise on best practices, fund critical action, and defend Uruguay's tobacco control policies.

The FCTC process, in particular, provided a basis for immediate action in the country and a blueprint for the types of policies that needed to be adopted. In one decade, Uruguay changed from a country in which tobacco control policies were limited and ineffective to a global example of the benefits resulting from FCTC implementation. Today, members of the Uruguayan tobacco control community serve as international leaders and mentors in their own right, helping other countries fulfill their FCTC commitments.

Much has been made of President Vázquez's exceptional leadership in implementing tobacco control initiatives in Uruguay and, indeed, it is difficult to imagine similar progress being achieved had he not been elected in late 2004. However, his leadership was driven by a committed group of advocates that fought hard to prepare the country for change. Moreover, the fact that every presidential decree has been incorporated, and in many cases even strengthened, into national law is a testament to the power and depth of the tobacco control community in Uruguay and its ability to use the FCTC to educate policymakers and change their perspectives on controlling tobacco.

At the same time, PMI's trade suit has sent a strong message to other low- and middle-income countries regarding the potential costs of passing effective tobacco control legislation. The final outcome of the case will redefine the relationship between trade and health and the future of tobacco control in the post-FCTC world.

CHAPTER SEVEN

The FCTC in Germany

An Island of Resistance

Throughout the negotiations for the Framework Convention on Tobacco Control, Germany was infamous for its opposition to a strong treaty. Along with the United States, China, and Japan, Germany fought to weaken obligations contained in the convention and consistently acted to protect tobacco industry interests.[1,2] Germany's position toward the FCTC came as no surprise and reflected its longstanding resistance to tobacco control. In 2002, in the midst of the FCTC negotiations, tobacco control activist David Simpson described tobacco control in Germany as "eerily reminiscent of the early days in the USA or the UK: the enemy seems all powerful, the press appears to believe every word they say, and the general public does not seem concerned either way."[3] Tobacco industry documents reveal that Germany was identified very early on in the FCTC process as a key target and potential ally in the industry's global strategy against the convention.[4] Party to the treaty since 2005, Germany has largely failed to pass any legislation relevant to its implementation.

Germany's scientific, political, and social attitudes toward tobacco have influenced how it has approached the FCTC and how it has impacted the global process. Although Germany's Nazi heritage and weak public health infrastructure have been linked to its pro-tobacco stance in the past, longstanding tobacco industry influence on science and policy has made the largest contribution to its resistance to the normative shifts regarding tobacco use and control taking place all around it.[5] Germany provides a difficult test case for the FCTC and illustrates how non-adopters of global public health norms can undermine global efforts and stall implementation. However, it also illustrates that no country is completely isolated from the activities taking place around it, and that international processes can make inroads at multiple levels, including academia, policymaking, and public opinion.

Pre-FCTC Germany

In the early twentieth century, Germany led the world in tobacco-related science. In 1909, German scientists first coined the term "secondhand smoke,"[6] and in 1929, Fritz Lickint published the first formal statistical evidence linking tobacco and lung cancer.[7] German scientists continued to make significant contributions to the tobacco and health evidence base throughout the 1930s, thanks to a substantial investment in cancer research by the Weimer Republic and the Nazi regime. During this time, the Nazi doctrine of "social hygiene" was implemented for the sake of "racial health."[8] Specifically, the regime focused on cancer prevention and initiated national campaigns against the hazards of smoking.[9] Smoking was presented as an "un-German habit" and as hazardous to the German "social body."[10] The Nazi government also issued sanctions against smokers, prohibited smoking in hospitals and public offices, demarcated special compartments for nonsmokers in trains, and restricted certain forms of cigarette advertising.[11] Despite these control efforts, smoking during the war years was pervasive (80% of German men smoked) and continued to increase. At the end of the war, the newly created West Germany was an easy target for a massive invasion by American tobacco companies. Against the backdrop of a country in ruins and a destroyed economy, imported cigarettes, notably Camels, were used on the black market in lieu of the inflated official currency.[12] Germans widely considered smoking to be one of the basic human needs, and they idealized it as "the last tiny bit of dignified life."[13]

Tobacco Industry Structure and Activities

It was at this time that the modern German tobacco industry began to take shape. The Verband der Cigarettenindustrie (VdC), the German trade association of cigarette manufacturers, was founded in 1948. Between 1954 and 2007, the VdC comprised German and Austrian tobacco companies (Reemtsma, Brinkmann, H. van Landewyck, Austria Tabak, and three smaller companies) as well as the German branches of three transnational firms (Philip Morris, RJ Reynolds, and British American Tobacco). Until its dissolution in 2007, the VdC had five departments: industrial activities, trade issues, marketing, public affairs, and the scientific department.[14,15] Unlike in the United States, where the industry split its political and scientific activities into separate organizations, the VdC was responsible for representing the companies' political interests and influencing the scientific community.[16]

Much of what is known about the activities of the VdC and transnational tobacco companies in Germany over the past half century comes from the tobacco
industry's own confidential documents released to the public as a result of litigation in the United States. The documents detail decades of scientific manipu-
lation and public deceit. The VdC's first scientific activities began in the early to
mid-1950s as evidence that cigarettes caused death and disease began to accumulate.[17,18] In the 1960s, transnational (primarily American) firms began actively
supporting the VdC's research in Germany.[19] American companies were particularly interested in their ability to use the VdC structure to conduct research at
an arm's length, thereby protecting themselves from litigation.[20]

The VdC and transnationals established a number of institutions through
which industry-supported research could be conducted and disseminated. The
VdC's scientific department was composed of industry representatives who dealt
with research projects funded by transnational and national tobacco companies.[21] The department was responsible for research that the industry did not
trust to be completed outside of the company. Between 1977 and 1999, the VdC
directly funded 110 research projects (most dealing with secondhand smoke) at
a total cost of more than $9.2 million.[22]

The VdC also established the semi-independent German Cigarette Research
Institute. It dismantled the institute in 1975 after its director, Professor Walter
Dontenwill, published an article in 1973 in the prestigious *Journal of the National
Cancer Institute* demonstrating that hamsters developed tumors of the larynx
after inhaling cigarette smoke.[23] After closing the institute, the VdC established
the Research Council on Smoking and Health in 1975 (renamed the Foundation
for Behavior and Environment in 1992). Although the first bylaws implied that
the council would be relatively independent, its role appears to have been limited
to recommending to the VdC which research should be funded.[24]

In addition to the scientific institutions funded collaboratively through the
VdC, transnational companies made use of their own research institutions in
Germany. This type of external research took place in several countries, but
Germany became home to the most developed scientific program supported by
transnational companies outside of the United States.[25,26] The VdC also paid
many researchers in independent academic institutions to conduct research that
more often than not resulted in favorable evidence for the industry. Throughout
the 1970s, the VdC and the transnational tobacco companies established a complex scientific network composed of individual scientists in Germany. The sheer
number of scientists collaborating with the tobacco industry in Germany and,
in some cases, the intensity of their involvement is remarkable in comparison to

scientists in other countries.[27] It was far less problematic for Germany and other countries to accept tobacco industry funding in the 1960s and 1970s than it was in later decades.[28] Perhaps even as late as the early 1980s, some German scientists may not have realized the implications of accepting industry funding, or that they would be working in a system so tightly controlled by an industry that was assuring them—often falsely—that they would have full independence. While the scientific community elsewhere in the world grew to reject tobacco industry funding and sought to mitigate its influence on science, many German scientists failed to do so.[29,30]

Although the tobacco industry carried out similar activities in a number of countries, the extent of the industry's success with conducting scientific research in Germany and influencing German scientific and public opinion was unparalleled.[31] Throughout the 1970s, 1980s, and even 1990s, the consumption of tobacco products in Germany was regarded as a "private sin," "harmless pleasure," or, at worst, an annoyance to non-smokers due to the lack of supposed scientific consensus on the health effects of active and passive smoking.[32] Consequently, the German public remains more smoker friendly than other high-income European countries and the United States and, after decades of steady decline, the consumption of tobacco products in Germany increased by 7.5% from 1996 to 2000.[33]

Control Efforts

The German healthcare system was radically reorganized in the late 1940s in response to its misuse during the Third Reich. The system was defined by decentralization, and any measures echoing the notion of a legal duty to preserve one's health were avoided. Public health prevention campaigns were considered too costly and inefficient, and tobacco control in particular was closely associated with taboos of the past.[34] When the first landmark studies linking smoking and lung cancer were released in 1950, many German doctors saw the whole area of research as "a poisoned chalice."[35]

It wasn't until the 1990s that public health became a recognized specialty in German medicine.[36] The first school of public health in the German-speaking region of Europe opened at Bielefeld University in 1994. Reflecting back on his time as the first chair of the university's Department of Public Health Medicine, Alexander Krämer noted that he and his colleagues "faced severe opposition from faculty, the university administration, and particularly reviewers of public health research grants" when pushing for tobacco prevention programs. These obstructions, Krämer argued, signaled that as of the mid-1990s, doctors and public health professionals in Germany were not yet ready to recognize the need to fight smoking.[37]

There were, however, some early legislative efforts to control smoking in Germany. Advertising was banned on television and radio in 1975, and health warnings, albeit weak ones, were required beginning in 1983. In regard to secondhand smoke, the German government identified the protection of non-smokers in public places as an urgent issue as early as May 1974.[38] The government argued at the time that "although the data on the real danger of 'passive smoking' is insufficient as of yet, a conclusion by analogy must be permitted that this danger is real" and that "it would be irresponsible to wait until a 'rash' of sick persons, people incapable of working and dead can be exhibited that fell victim to passive smoking."[39] In response, members of the Bundestag (lower house of the German parliament) passed a resolution calling on the federal government to prepare a comprehensive program for the protection of non-smokers. However, when the German government finally released a program in 1978, it argued: "Any governmental intervention limiting the citizen's rights to develop his own personality in the form of general bans are only justified in restricted areas. A general ban on smoking, however, is not in line with the appropriateness of means. The smoker's and nonsmokers personal rights should be weighed against one another."[40] In response to the non-binding recommendations outlined in the program, the government did not propose any new legislation or additional financial resources for the protection of non-smokers. The government's reversal can be accredited to the initiation of a massive campaign of persuading German politicians undertaken by the tobacco industry at the time.[41]

Following the 1978 program, the German government did not formally address comprehensive tobacco control again until 1990. The revised government program was developed partially in response to the 1986 US Surgeon General's Report, which concluded that secondhand smoke caused lung cancer in adults. The 1990 program, however, did not represent a substantial step forward from the 1978 program. It consisted of an educational campaign targeted at adolescents and made some recommendations on tobacco cessation, self-regulation of access to tobacco products, protection of non-smokers, tobacco advertising, and warning labels.[42] Even the weak recommendations did not specify who would be responsible for implementation. Minutes of a VdC board meeting in August 1990 once again accredited the industry for considerably weakening earlier drafts of the 1990 program, including completely removing recommended tax increases and provisions to limit easy access to tobacco products.[43]

In 1994, 41 members of the Bundestag once again proposed a draft bill for federal legislation aimed at protecting non-smokers. The proposed bill received extensive negative press. Less than one month before the final parliamentary vote, a major German newspaper (*Frankfurter Allgemeine Zeitung*) reported on a study that found the potential cost to German businesses of a law to protect against smoking to be $16 billion.[44] The study was carried out by an independent economic research institute, but commissioned by the tobacco industry. Another industry study covered extensively in the press reported that more than three-quarters of Germans did not want new legislation on secondhand smoke.[45] The German Nonsmokers Initiative, a network of German tobacco control NGOs, did release a press statement highlighting the industry's ties to these studies and suggesting that the poll results were in stark contrast with all relevant surveys.[46] However, the press release failed to garner any attention from media outlets. On February 5, 1998, the federal non-smoker protection legislation was defeated. After two other failed attempts at passing a comprehensive non-smoker protection bill, a weak ordinance nominally providing workplace protection was passed in 2001. At a VdC Science and Industry Policy Committee meeting in 2002, VdC representatives expressed pleasure that secondhand smoke was once again no longer a pressing topic in Germany.[47]

Civil Society and the Courts

The industry's influence on German policymakers and the public was especially great because of the lack of other credible sources of tobacco information. Non-governmental health organizations in Germany did not continuously prioritize tobacco control. One exception was the Medical Action Group on Smoking or Health, which was founded in 1971 by Ferdinand Schmidt, a medical scientist and director of the Research Center for Preventive Oncology in Mannheim. In 1972, the Medical Action Group called for statutory protection of non-smokers in its program against smoking, and it organized the first German Nonsmokers Conference in 1974.[48] The tobacco industry responded to the group's activities by framing the work of Schmidt as "peculiar."[49] The industry attacks continued into the 1990s and were successful at marginalizing Schmidt in the eyes of scientists and government health administrators.[50] The German Nonsmokers Initiative was another non-governmental organization established in 1988 to unite local and regional groups fighting for smoke-free workplaces. The largest member of the network was the Munich chapter, which had been sued in 1984 by Philip Morris for its use of the Marlboro Poker campaign as a basis for their "Death Poker" (in

German, *Mordoro Poker*) campaign in which the prizes were advertised as lung cancer and heart attacks. In this case the Federal Court of Justice in Germany ruled in favor of the NGO.

This was not the only example of German courts' early engagement in tobacco control. Beginning in the early 1980s, numerous law review articles and court decisions accompanied the growing awareness of the hazards of smoking, and these sources testify to at least some tobacco control activism in the German legal class.[51] In a series of decisions, courts (mainly labor courts) issued injunctions against smoking in the workplace.[52] These cases largely originated from state-level laws adopted in the late 1970s that gave non-smokers the freedom to insist that their employers take action to prevent detrimental health effects related to tobacco. The typical situation involved employees going to court after management failed to meet their demands for smoke-free areas.[53] By 1994, roughly 60 courts had decided in favor of the plaintiffs based on either labor or civil service law.[54] In 1998, the Federal Labor Court decided that workers and employees are entitled to a "tobacco-free" workplace if so required by reasons of health; for example, because they suffer from pulmonary disease.[55] However, the 1998 Federal Labor Court decision depends on the willingness of non-smokers to defend their health in court—leaving them open to retaliation by their employers.

Although the courts provided an important ally in German tobacco control efforts, there was no significant tobacco litigation in Germany similar to that in the United States. This difference may be due less to differences in liability law than to the fact that smoking-related health costs are covered by health insurance in Germany.[56] Hence, smokers can't go to court and sue a tobacco company for medical costs that were covered by state insurance companies. German insurance companies have been reluctant to litigate because, in addition to public health insurance, they also provide old-age insurance. To argue financial loss associated with tobacco use, they would have to show proof that, on balance, the smoking-related health costs are not compensated by a reduction in their payouts for health and social security pension insurance.[57]

European Union Attempts to Regulate Tobacco

Since the early 1970s, the European Union has attempted to exert control over tobacco in its member states. Early EU efforts focused on harmonizing tobacco taxes throughout the market. These efforts were met with a great deal of resistance from many member states, including Germany, which feared being deprived of a crucial source of income.[58] However, in subsequent years, Germany has often stood alone in its refusal to accept EU promotion of tobacco control policies throughout the region.

The first case in which Germany aggressively tried to stop EU regulation of tobacco came in 1989, when the EU passed a directive requiring that specific health warnings—such as "Cigarette smoking is hazardous to your health" and "Smoking causes cancer"—be included on all cigarette packages and advertisements. The tobacco industry challenged the EU directive in the German Federal Constitutional Court, arguing that the legally required warnings were violations of the tobacco companies' constitutionally protected commercial speech, which emanated from freedom of speech under the Basic Law for the Federal Republic of Germany.[59] During the period leading up to the court's decision, politicians, legal scholars, and the tobacco industry criticized the EU directive for restating the opinion of cancer experts who based their judgment on "questionable statistical" data provided primarily by the US surgeon gSeneral.[60,61] In addition, the controversy concentrated on the EU's competence to take regulatory action in the field of health policy under the guise of harmonizing the national regulations governing the labels for tobacco products, and on the negative freedoms of commercial speech.[62] During debate at the European Commission, the German minister of health pushed to modify the warnings by including the word "may" in "Smoking causes cancer." The commission rejected the intervention, emphatically stating that such a conditional modification was scientifically incorrect.

In 1997, the German Federal Constitutional Court finally confirmed the conditionality of the aforementioned warnings.[63] However, based on the German case, national and EU ministers of public health did revise the warnings to clarify that the ministers, not the companies, were the authors. EU law regarding cigarette packages was further strengthened in 2003. In each instance, Germany was forced to implement stronger health warnings because of formal harmonization, and not due to independent decision-making.

The tobacco industry's use of the German Federal Constitutional Court in the health warnings case was largely viewed as a test for the impending battle over an EU-wide comprehensive advertising and sponsorship ban. The idea of such a ban was first proposed in 1989, at which point the industry reasoned that should the labeling directive conflict with the German constitution, the health warnings lawsuit could be used to challenge the main elements of any future EU advertising ban. As early as 1990, the industry was also developing plans to challenge such a ban at the supranational level through the European Court of Justice (ECJ), with the anticipation that Germany would bring such a case on the industry's behalf.[64]

In 1992, the European Parliament voted to impose the advertising and sponsorship ban despite massive lobbying by the tobacco and advertising industries. The comprehensive ban was intended to standardize the EU as a single market for tobacco advertising. However, progress on the bill stalled in the Council of Ministers, where the ban was subject to a qualified majority, enabling a small number of countries to block it. Between 1992 and 1995, no qualified majority was possible; naturally, Germany was among those voting to block the bill (along with The Netherlands and the United Kingdom).[65]

During its period of EU presidency in 1995, Germany attempted to introduce an amended bill, which was widely suspected at the time (and subsequently confirmed by industry documents) to have been developed by the industry. The bill stipulated that minimum advertising restrictions agreed on by all EU members would be set forth in the directive, and that member states would then be free to introduce more stringent restrictions.[66] The bill, which would have had little impact on countries with weak tobacco control policies, failed to get adequate support. The deadlock in the Council of Ministers was finally overcome after the UK position changed with the election of a Labor government in 1997, and in May 1998, the European Parliament ratified the directive with no amendments. Most German members, with the exception of the Green party, voted against the directive.[67]

In September 1998, just before Chancellor Helmut Kohl's term in office expired, Germany and four British tobacco companies filed suit before the ECJ, arguing that the directive was illegal. Specifically, the German government claimed that the directive violated the rights of tobacco manufacturers and advertising agencies under EU primary law, notably the European Community Treaty, by restricting free trade and the free flow of services.[68] The German government also argued that the EU acted outside its area of competence because article 129 of the EC Treaty expressly excludes the ability to take harmonizing measures for public health purposes. The ECJ's advocate general supported the German government's position in relation to the legal basis and proportionality of the directive and concluded that the directive had exceeded its legal basis as an internal market measure. The ECJ upheld the challenge and rescinded the advertising directive in November 2000.[69] Germany's focus on resisting EU and other external influence on tobacco control would extend to its participation in the coming FCTC negotiations.

The FCTC Process in Germany

Germany's resistance to the FCTC process began as early as 1996, when it voted against initiating work on the convention (World Health Assembly resolution 49.17). At the 1998 World Health Assembly, Germany described the proposed convention as "an unnecessary distraction from the work of WHO and not likely to be very effective." During the first working group meeting, the German delegation was mostly silent, although it did stress the possible negative economic consequences of tobacco control and the need for an economic impact study by the time of the second working group meeting. Germany included a representative from the Federal Ministry of the Economy on its delegation, making it one of the few countries to send a non-health representative at this point in the process. At the second working group meeting, Germany argued that as many member states as possible should agree to the principles of the framework convention, asserting that flexibility in the text was a condition of success.

Recognizing the need to put greater pressure on Germany to support the FCTC process, Derek Yach, then director of WHO's Tobacco Free Initiative (TFI), visited Hannover, Germany in August 2000 and gave a speech coinciding with the city's hosting of Expo 2000 (the World's Fair). Against the advice of many who feared that it would upset the German government, Yach spoke passionately about Germany's poor record in tobacco control and called on the country to "recognize that tobacco companies operate in a sphere that is outside the realm of the acceptable."[70] The message, however, failed to influence Germany's approach.

Negotiating Positions

As the negotiations went on, Germany developed more specific arguments against key elements of the treaty, particularly in regard to advertising restrictions, youth access, and language prioritizing free trade before health.[71] In 2000, the German Advertising Federation (of which the VdC was a member) claimed that a total advertising ban would be unconstitutional. Germany subsequently took the lead, along with the United States, in opposing comprehensive bans on advertising, promotion, and sponsorship.[72] In regard to youth access, Germany joined Japan in opposing bans on vending machines, arguing instead for the installation of age verification systems. Other countries grew so frustrated with this approach that the final FCTC text, although not requiring a ban on vending machines, allows countries to declare when signing the treaty that they intend to follow through with a complete ban. Germany also joined the United States and Japan in arguing unsuccessfully for prioritizing trade over health in the language of the convention.

Germany was also effective in forcing the EU to oppose many obligations it might have otherwise supported. Under EU law, member states can authorize the European Commission to negotiate and sign international agreements on their behalf in areas where policy is already covered by EU treaties. The EU generally has exclusive competence in areas where it has already legislated (e.g., tar yields and tobacco product labeling); in other areas, competence is either shared among the EU and member states (e.g., tax or tobacco advertising) or member states have exclusive competence (vending machines, smoke-free public places). To simplify this complex situation, the EU and member states agreed on two negotiating mandates in October 1999 and April 2001. Although these agreements were not made public, confidential industry documents confirm that Germany was key in limiting the scope of the mandates to labeling and cigarette contents and excluding fiscal and agricultural issues. Consequently, during the negotiations the European Commission negotiated on behalf of the EU member states in areas where it had exclusive competence (labeling), whereas the country holding the presidency negotiated in areas of shared competence and exclusive member states' competence. Germany's positions throughout the negotiations won it four Dirty Ashtray Awards from the Framework Convention Alliance (it came in third place after the United States and Japan for number of awards), including one for "dragging down the entire European region to the level of the USA."[73]

Tobacco Industry Influence

There is concrete evidence that Germany's positions toward the FCTC were highly influenced by the tobacco industry. According to previously confidential tobacco industry documents, Germany was targeted early on due to its close links and established resistance to tobacco control, influence on the international system, and prominent role in WHO and the FCTC process. Germany's influence on the FCTC process was especially great given its representation on the WHO executive board and on the FCTC working groups. Mr. Helmut Voigtländer, director of EU affairs at the German Federal Health Ministry (FHM), represented Germany in both these forums. In 1999, when speaking to what he thought was a journalist investigating an article on WHO tobacco policies, but who was actually an undercover industry public relations lead, Mr. Voigtländer said that he thought the convention should be kept "very broad," he did not believe in "radical" tobacco control measures such as price increases or advertising bans, and he could anticipate working with the tobacco industry. Such comments raised the tobacco industry's confidence in using Germany as its key agenda-weakening state. The industry's influence on German policy was enhanced through close relationships among VdC board members, the German Chancellery, and the Federal Ministry of Health throughout the process.

Evidence suggests that the industry undermined the federal health minister's position by creating controversy among financial, trade, and other ministries while business associations and other front groups lobbied on the industry's behalf. For example, the VdC successfully stymied the FHM's plan to wait to hold the first inter-ministerial consultation until after the first working group by having other federal ministers insist that the consultation take place beforehand. According to industry documents, this meeting held just before the first working group consisted of a very controversial debate between the different federal ministries, during which the FHM representatives were surprised to learn about the other ministries' opposition to the FCTC. Against the wishes of the FHM, the ministries decided at this meeting that Germany should only support initiatives on health information and education, labeling, and cigarette content, and should not agree to other proposals, such as those on testing methods, smuggling, prices, taxes, and advertising.

The tobacco industry also took advantage of Germany's link to the International Standard Organization (ISO) to influence the FCTC negotiations. In 1999, WHO sought membership in ISO's technical committee 126 on tobacco products and testing methodologies, which was run by the German Institute for Standardization (DIN). DIN, which included tobacco industry employees on its committee on tobacco smoke, used WHO's application to insist that ISO committee representatives be allowed to participate in WHO tobacco-related activities as an organization in "official relations." This designation was traditionally used by WHO to facilitate pro–tobacco control civil society organizations' access to WHO processes. However, as a consequence of WHO's agreement with ISO, German tobacco industry employees gained access to working group meetings and the first four intergovernmental negotiating bodies (INBs) as observers representing ISO.

Other private sector interests outside the tobacco industry also influenced Germany's anti-FCTC stance. Four industry umbrella groups (German Wholesale and Foreign Trade, German Association of Chambers of Industry and Commerce, Foreign Trade Association of the German Retail Trade, and Federation of German Industries) all testified during WHO's public hearings in support of standard tobacco industry arguments and continued to oppose the treaty throughout the remainder of the process.

Ratification

At the end of the FCTC negotiations in February 2003, Germany (along with the United States) opposed the treaty's final text, arguing that the German constitution prevented it from introducing a comprehensive ban on tobacco advertising, promotion, and sponsorship. Until the very last minute of debate, other EU countries believed the only way to overcome German opposition to the treaty was to introduce reservations to the treaty (something that other countries refused to allow). However, hours before the start of the World Health Assembly, a German official announced in Geneva that Berlin had decided not to challenge the agreement. As explained previously, the reasons for the German/US turnaround are unknown and cause for much speculation.

On December 16, 2004, Germany ratified the FCTC, making it just short of being in the initial group of 40 ratifications required to make the treaty enter into force. After ratification, the German government initially failed to prepare legislation relevant to the implementation of the FCTC. By ratifying, the issue was effectively neutralized. Tobacco control advocates could no longer launch an aggressive mass media campaign pushing for ratification, and the Ministry of Health publically argued that everything required by the FCTC was already in place in Germany.[74] In fact, the only area in which Germany was in compliance was with the 30% health warning labels that were in place as a consequence of the 2001 EU regulation.

Post-FCTC Tobacco Control in Germany

German resistance to tobacco control efforts continued following its formal commitment to the FCTC. A 2006 survey of tobacco control activities ranked Germany last in tobacco control in Europe. This ranking included last place in scientific research on tobacco-related issues, healthcare involvement in tobacco control, protection from secondhand smoke, taxation, political will to enact tobacco control measures, media support for tobacco control, and population support for tobacco control.

When the German government changed hands in late 2005, there was some hope that Chancellor Angela Merkel would be more supportive of efforts to con-

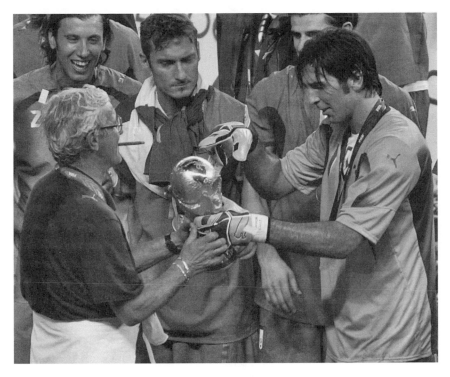

Figure 14. Italy's coach Marcello Lippi (left) holds the trophy with goalkeeper Gian-luigi Buffon after defeating France 5–3 in a shootout in the 2006 World Cup final held in Berlin. Associated Press Photo / Michael Probst

trol tobacco than her predecessors. Merkel is a scientist and appears to take sci-entific evidence much more seriously than past chancellors. However, the Merkel coalition government did not show increased political will for tobacco control.

One example of Germany's ongoing resistance to global efforts to address to-bacco under Merkel's leadership came when Germany hosted the World Cup in 2006. In 2002, the World Cup host countries, Japan and South Korea (both to-bacco control resistors themselves) agreed with the Fédération Internationale de Football Association (FIFA) and WHO on a memorandum of understanding for a smoke-free World Cup. Smoking was banned in stadiums, and no official to-bacco advertising and merchandise were permitted in association with the tour-nament. When WHO, FIFA, and public health groups approached the German officials before the 2006 World Cup, they were informed that Germany would not renew the memorandum of understanding.[75] Despite a late effort by national and international public health groups to pressure the German officials to change their policy, smoking was permitted in the stadiums and on the fields during the 2006 World Cup. Moreover, ashtrays and other tobacco-related official merchandise were sold. Images of smoking fans and coaches were commonly seen on television throughout the tournament—including one of the Italian coach smoking as he accepted the trophy at the end of the tournament.

Also in 2006, Germany's deadline to incorporate the 2003 EU Tobacco Advertising Directive into national law passed without Merkel's government making any attempt to prepare the needed legislation. The new directive was considerably weakened from the 2000 version, confining itself to issues of cross-border advertising (in print media and on the radio and internet) and sponsorship. Heeding the ECJ ruling, the new draft directive omitted the usual safeguard clause and the ban on indirect advertising, which was specifically mentioned by the advocate general as having an unproven impact on consumption. The European Parliament approved the new directive in 2003 and, once again, Germany issued a challenge in the ECJ. In June, after the ECJ's advocate general recommended a dismissal of the case, German lawmakers finally submitted a bill to parliament banning tobacco advertising.[76] At the time, the lawmakers argued that the legal basis for the directive was correct, and that Germany was facing fines of up to €110,000 per day starting in 2007. German Consumer Protection Minister Horst Seehofer also announced that his government would give in to the growing pressure from the ECJ to ban tobacco advertising, arguing that the government challenge to the ban was due to concern for the rights of EU member states to maintain sovereignty over certain areas of law, and not by any strong objection to the ban itself.[77] In December 2006, an advertising ban for print and online media based on the EU directive entered into force in Germany. The partial ban still fell far below the bans on advertising, sponsorship, and promotion called for in the FCTC.

Legislative Changes Since 2006

Inspired by the success of smoke-free legislation in neighboring European countries, two groups of parliamentarians made independent proposals for comprehensive smoke-free legislation in 2006. The bills caught the attention of the press, and the government was put under pressure to take some form of action. The grand coalition government established a working group to consider the issue and to draft a comprehensive law. The tobacco industry's influence over the working group, however, was so apparent that the group was labeled an industry "puppet" by the media. Not only was the text of the law severely weakened, with pubs and bars totally excluded and restaurants partially exempted, but media reports also uncovered how text citing a VdC position paper verbatim found its way into the draft.[78] During the working group discussions, the justice department sent a memo to the working group informing them that any ban on specific venues was outside the jurisdiction of the federal government.[79] The only legal approach that the working group could take was to recommend a complete ban in all workplaces under federal workplace safety legislation.

The legislation finally recommended by the group in December 2006 was comparatively weak; it still allowed smoking in bars, pubs, and enclosed smoking rooms in restaurants. Nevertheless, it was highly controversial in a country that had always favored industry self-regulation. Within days, government leaders, including Chancellor Merkel, expressed concern that national legislation to protect the public from secondhand smoke was unconstitutional and that jurisdiction to regulate restaurants fell to the states.[80] Whereas the FMH argued that the constitution allows the federal government to take measures against public health risks, the federal ministries of justice and internal affairs countered that the law required such health risks to represent an immediate danger to the public and thus did not cover smoking. On this subject, the media consistently quoted Rupert Scholz, university professor of law and former minister of defense and member of parliament. What was not mentioned in any of the media reports at the time was the longstanding link between Scholz and the German tobacco industry. In the 1990s, for example, Scholz was vice chair of a research institute established and financed by the tobacco industry, and Scholz continued to serve on its board in 2007. A scaled-back version of the law eventually entered into force in 2007 that banned smoking in federal buildings, public transport, and train stations.

The failure to pass comprehensive smoke-free legislation at the national level forced German states to address the issue. Between August 2007 and January 2008, laws were passed in 16 states banning smoking in local authority buildings, educational institutions, and hospitals, and restricting smoking in restaurants and bars. Each state faces its own challenges in passing and enforcing smoking bans, and many continue to fight to close loopholes that allow smokers to continue to smoke inside. Bavaria, for example, passed its law in January 2008, but the law failed to contain provisions for ensuring compliance, and smoking was once again permitted in small bars and in secondary rooms of other hospitality premises later that year. At the end of 2009, many Bavarian institutions, including opposition political parties, medical organizations, non-smokers' groups, and sports associations, supported a petition in favor of a referendum for a smoking ban without exemptions. Within two weeks, 1.3 million Bavarian voters signed the petition, far surpassing the required 10%.

The tobacco industry countered the referendum (held July 4, 2010) with a massive public relations campaign. A strategic alliance was set up that consisted of the tobacco industry, the brewery trade, the hospitality industry, advertising agencies, and slot machine operators. The main campaign message was that a smoke-free hospitality industry would lead to mass bankruptcy and the loss of freedom and tolerance. Millions of posters and flyers proclaimed "Bavaria says NO!" and tobacconists distributed more than 1.6 million cigarette lighters for free, with combative slogans such as "Who sleeps in democracy will wake up in dictatorship." Both sides mobilized their support via the internet, including through Facebook, which led to a sustained radicalism among many bar owners and smokers. The spokesperson of the Alliance for the Protection of Non-Smokers was called a Nazi and received death threats. The massive industry financial investment and political pressure used in the campaign backfired when the public gained insight into their tactics and influence. The referendum ended with a clear public vote of 61% in favor of a complete smoking ban in the hospitality industry, and smoking has been banned in Bavarian bars, restaurants, and beer tents since August 1, 2010.

Persisting Tobacco Industry Influence

Although the story from Bavaria testifies to growing public intolerance of the tobacco industry, the inability to pass effective tobacco control legislation at the federal level illustrates the continued influence of the tobacco industry on the German political establishment. This influence can be linked to its ongoing financial support of the political system through direct lobbying and support for political events and specific programs. Shortly before the release of the comprehensive smoke-free legislation in 2006, for example, Philip Morris co-sponsored the annual convention of the Christian Democratic Union, the political party of Chancellor Merkel. The VdC, Philip Morris, and Reestma officially donated more than €300,000 to the Free Democratic Party, Social Democratic Party, and Christian Democratic Union in the years 1997 to 2003. The extent of additional donations to individual politicians is unknown. Even the Green Party has been tainted by tobacco funding.

The German government fails to recognize problems arising from accepting tobacco industry money. For example, in 2002 the German government made an agreement with the Association of Tobacco Industry in which the industry provided €11.8 million for a five-year tobacco control program purporting to prevent children and adolescents from smoking. According to the contract, the industry supposedly had no influence on the content or style of the campaigns, but the "measures must not discriminate against the tobacco industry, its products and the sale of cigarettes, or criticize adult smokers."[81] The resulting campaign from the FMH, "RauchFrei" (Smoke Free), comprised posters showing attractive young people smoking, accompanied by big slogans such as "Smoking soothes" and "Smoking makes you adult," with statements in smaller type such as "Right: but with carcinogenic substances such as arsenic, radon, or tar." The campaign quickly became an international scandal. John Seffrin, president of the Union for International Cancer Control (UICC), said it was "despicable that a government should take money from tobacco companies that dictate the conditions of an anti-smoking campaign."[82] German Cancer Aid, the leading German cancer charity, asked the German health ministry to stop the anti-smoking advertisements immediately. Numerous letters were written in prominent international journals criticizing the agreement.[83,84] The German government, however, has continued to defend its contract with the industry, arguing that the national prevention program aims to make non-smoking a national norm.[85] Additional non-industry–supported expenditures for anti-tobacco campaigns have been low from the government.

With few exceptions, most tobacco control measures in Germany remain largely voluntary in nature, adopted by the tobacco industry to prevent formal legislation. Their implementation is often weak and even nonexistent. Youth access to tobacco is one example of such measures. There are more than 800,000 cigarette vending machines in Germany—one for every 30 smokers.[86] Traditionally, these machines have been located in unsecured locations. A study conducted in 2005 found that 60.7% of all cigarette vending machines were located in areas where there was little to no control of youth access.[87] Vending machines became a major political issue when new measures were launched in 2001 after reports revealed that 28% of German youth were active smokers. Efforts to curb street vending machines, however, were strongly challenged by the industry. Eventually, a compromise was reached between the German government and the industry: to buy a pack of cigarettes from a vending machine, an adult smoker must use a debit card embedded with a microchip that contains a youth protection symbol.[88] By January 1, 2007, all cigarette machines were required to have chip cards. The 2007 law also required that all cigarette packages have at least 19 cig-

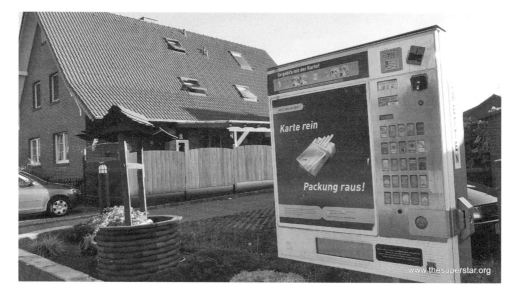

Figure 15. "Card In, Pack Out": Cigarette vending machine in Germany that requires an identity card for purchases. http://www.superstar.org (used under CC BY-ND 2.0)

arettes, and it raised the legal age to purchase tobacco and legally smoke in public from 16 to 18, although there was a two-year transition phase enabling vending machine purchases by youth ages 16–18 until 2009.

Despite the weakness of the revised youth access laws, youth smoking decreased between 2001 and 2008. This decrease is likely a consequence of Germany's multiple tobacco tax increases since 2000. Between 2002 and 2010, the average tobacco tax increased by 75%.[89]

Scientific and Civil Society Engagement

The scientific community in Germany continues to lack a code of ethics regarding tobacco industry funding disclaimers.[90] However, it has grown increasingly difficult for German scientists to publish research studies that challenge the scientific status quo regarding active and passive smoking.[91] As recently as 2000, top medical journals in Germany published studies that showed no association between secondhand smoke and disease. However, outrage among some medical professionals expressed in letters to the editors appears to have convinced journal editors that such studies should no longer be accepted for publication.[92] There also has been increased media scrutiny of scientists who work closely with the tobacco industry. In 2005, the popular news magazine *Der Spiegel* published a lengthy article about the industry's influence on science and scientists in Germany, specifically naming a number of scientists found in industry documents.[93] Although the scientists identified in the article denied industry influence on their work, two were forced to resign from their posts.[94] Still, the Philip Morris Science Award continues to be popular in Germany, and many members of the German scientific community continue to accept tobacco industry support.[95] Many influential scientists also continue to sit on the board of the VdC.

The WHO Collaborating Center on Tobacco Control at the German Cancer Research Center in Heidelberg represents one major difference in the tobacco control environment in Germany since the start of the FCTC process.[96] The center conducts health-related research and provides a central focus for much of the tobacco control activities that now take place in Germany. It was established in 1999 at the start of the FCTC process after Derek Yach grew concerned that tobacco control allies were urgently needed in Germany. In addition to establishing the formal institutional relationship with the center, WHO invited its leader, Dr. Martina Poetschke-Langer, to participate in the Tobacco Free Initiative's program aimed at developing national tobacco control leaders and agents of change. Consequently, WHO sent Dr. Poetschke-Langer to the University of California, San Francisco, to learn about California's successful efforts in reducing tobacco use and to Washington, DC, to work with Mike Pertschuk, the co-founder and co-director of the Advocacy Institute.

According to Dr. Poetschke-Langer, her time at the Advocacy Institute was a career-changing experience in which she finally realized the importance of policy and media advocacy.[97] Dr. Poetschke-Langer has used this new knowledge to develop personal contacts with members of the media, resulting in media coverage of industry influence and tobacco control in Germany. In 2006, for example, Dr. Poetschke-Langer convinced *Der Spiegel* to publish a 12-page article criticizing Germany's record in tobacco control.[98] The article outlined in detail the steps that were being taken in other European countries to control tobacco. The German position on tobacco at the 2006 World Cup was highly criticized in the magazine, which stated that even China, which was well known for weak tobacco control, had committed to making the 2008 Olympics smoke free.[99] In addition to her work with the media, Dr. Poetschke-Langer has established stronger links with legislators and was instrumental in convincing policymakers to introduce the secondhand smoke bills in 2006.

The German Cancer Research Center has joined the "RauchFrei" campaign and a small number of health agencies, including German Cancer Aid and other

German cancer societies, to form a national tobacco control coalition. Together, the coalition has undertaken limited political work; since 2005, they have paid for a full-time lobbyist in Berlin. Unfortunately, the coalition's effectiveness reportedly has been reduced by political in-fighting between the members and the lack of a coordinated approach. According to US tobacco control advocate John Bloom, the situation with the German coalition is reminiscent of the environment in the United States before the Campaign for Tobacco-Free Kids and the Legacy Foundation took active leads in advocating for tobacco control at the national level.[100]

Germany's approach to the FCTC was largely consistent with its historically weak tobacco control policies and repeated opposition to EU tobacco control legislation. Its positions reflected widespread influence of the tobacco industry on German policymaking. Germany is one of the few industrialized nations in which the tobacco industry remains a legitimate force in business, government, science, and society at large.[101] The industry's strategy to leverage Germany's position to affect the final outcomes of the FCTC was to some extent successful; the final convention includes text reflective of Germany's influence, including the allowances for countries to implement or decline bans on advertising, promotion, and sponsorship in accordance with their constitution or constitutional principles.

The FCTC conversely has had very little influence on domestic tobacco control in Germany. The federal government has refused to pursue a regulatory path that would provoke opposition from the tobacco industry and has denied federal efforts to enact extensive regulations. The political environment surrounding tobacco control in the federal government continues to demonstrate the tobacco industry's ability to influence politicians through promises of financial and political support or by threats of legal challenges and economic hardship. Although Germany has raised taxes, introduced minimal smoke-free legislation, and implemented some restrictions on advertising and cigarette sales to minors, these policies fail to meet the FCTC guidelines. Germany continues to be ranked among the most inactive European countries in terms of tobacco control policies, and the FCTC movement has not had an extensive impact on forming a strong social movement or viable and vocal coalition of groups and organizations. Tobacco control continues to be the concern of an enlightened few who come from the ranks of the medical profession, the state administration, and the legal profession.[102] Consequently, Germans continue to have one of the highest smoking rates in Europe, with 38.9% of German men and 30.6% of German women smoking. Even more troubling, 20.6% of German women continue to smoke during pregnancy.[103]

Nevertheless, regulatory and public change is taking place in Germany. Higher taxes and state smoking bans have started to reduce tobacco consumption, and four of five Germans now approve of protections for non-smokers.[104] The European Union has forced Germany to shift its stance on tobacco advertising and labeling, and if it continues to pursue a stricter course of action, public authorities in Germany may be forced to conform.[105] Tobacco control developments in the United States and other European countries are also carefully observed in Germany by both the defenders of the status quo and those who wish to change it. As the global norm of tobacco control is further diffused throughout the international system and confirmed by states and societies, Germany will be under increasing pressure to conform, even in the absence of formal harmonization or diffusion efforts by the European Union or WHO.

CHAPTER EIGHT

The FCTC in China

The "Responsible" Resistor

China is the world's largest tobacco market, accounting for 38% of the world's cigarette sales and one-third of the world's smokers.[1] With 320 million smokers (more than the entire US population) and one million premature deaths caused by smoking each year, China represents the largest single stakeholder in implementation of the Framework Convention on Tobacco Control (FCTC).[2] It also represents global tobacco control's greatest challenge.

Tobacco control in China is defined by significant conflicts of interest in the government. Although responsible for protecting the health of its citizens, the Chinese government is also the sole owner of the world's largest tobacco company, the China National Tobacco Corporation (CNTC), which is run by the State Tobacco Monopoly Association (STMA). The CNTC is responsible for growing, producing, marketing, distributing, and selling all tobacco products in China. In addition to this conflict of interest between the government's health imperative and its profitable tobacco business, the ruling party's ideology, the structure of domestic institutions, and the marginalized role of NGOs complicate tobacco control policymaking. Consequently, contradiction and largely opaque decision-making processes mark tobacco control in China.

China actively participated in the FCTC negotiations, during which it was known by international observers as one of the "Big Four" countries that effectively fought against strong commitments in the final FCTC text.[3] China's positions, however, were more nuanced than those of the other three countries (Japan, Germany, and the United States), reflecting its desire to be seen as a "responsible" country in line with international public health norms and its government's increasing awareness that certain elements of the FCTC could actually enhance governmental control of the domestic tobacco market. China ratified the FCTC in 2005, but it has largely failed to adopt domestic tobacco control legislation or implement relevant programs since the treaty entered into force in the country in January 2006. China's failure to internalize international tobacco control norms represents a major challenge to the FCTC's goals concerning global tobacco consumption and related mortality and morbidity.

The Pre-FCTC Tobacco Environment in China

In the mid-1990s, before the launch of the FCTC process, tobacco use was ubiquitous and widely accepted throughout China.[4] Results from the 1996 National Smoking Prevalence Study indicated that 63% of Chinese men and 3.8% of Chinese women smoked, only a minority of smokers were aware that smoking caused lung cancer (36%) and heart disease (4%), and very few smokers at the time had ever attempted quitting (approximately 6%). In addition, 53.5% of Chinese non-smokers were exposed to secondhand smoke for at least 15 minutes a day on more than one day per week.[5] Offering cigarettes was a common way to make an introduction or solidify a new friendship or business deal in China, and cigarettes were given as wedding gifts and even offered as thank-you gifts from patients to doctors. Declining a cigarette was often considered an insult. Many characters on television and film were heavy smokers, as were past political leaders, including Mao Zedong and Deng Xiaoping.

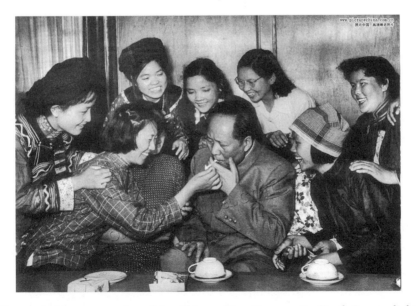

Figure 16. A representative of the Chinese New Democratic Youth League lights Chairman Mao Zedong's cigarette at the Third National Congress in 1957. Wikimedia Commons / People's Republic of China government

Tobacco control–related activities in China before the FCTC process were largely limited to research by health experts from national public health institutions. In the 1990s, for example, Dr. Gonghuan Yang, a 1982 graduate of Huaxi Medical University and 1987 visiting scholar at the Harvard School of Public Health, received funding and research support from foreign academic partners to perform several important surveys on tobacco prevalence in China. Based on these and other surveys, Chinese researchers estimated that more than 500,000 deaths per year were caused by smoking-related illnesses, and they projected that this number would rise to two million annual deaths by 2020.[6] This authoritative data on tobacco use in China served as a basis for increasingly strong calls to action.

The Chinese Association for Smoking and Health (CASH), the Chinese equivalent of a non-governmental organization, was formed in 1990 and established provisional branches throughout the country over the next ten years. The group helped to organize the annual National Symposium on Smoking and Health in China, which began in 1990 and, in 1997, had infamously grown into a literal "boatload" of tobacco control advocates, scientists, ministry of health officials, and teachers. With funding support from the Union for International Cancer Control (UICC), the small but dedicated group of domestic and international participants carried out the annual symposium while sailing up the Yangtze river for five days—signifying the upstream battle they faced against the tobacco epidemic in China.[7] Although a myriad of small-scale interventions, including legislation, regulations, and health education campaigns, were carried out in China in the 1990s, very little tobacco control progress was achieved. CASH's ability to aggressively advocate for policy change was complicated by the government's control over civil society and lack of tolerance for dissenting voices.

The lack of any significant progress in tobacco control before the FCTC (and since) can be directly linked to the national tobacco monopoly's economic and political influence on the Chinese government. In 2000, for example, research revealed that the annual cost of tobacco use in disease and death amounted to $5 billion, but profits and taxes from the government-run corporation amounted to more than ten times that amount.[8] The CNTC employed more than 500,000 workers in more than 180 factories, 150 tobacco-drying plants, and 30 research institutes. A total of ten million people (tobacco company workers, farmers, and shop owners) made a living from China's state-run tobacco industry.[9] Money from tobacco was the single largest source of revenue for the Chinese market, with some provinces (e.g., Yunnan province) totally dependent on money from tobacco to keep their governments running.[10] Although the CNTC essentially controlled all tobacco production in the country, local governments were responsible for implementing the production plan assigned by the state planning department and for assisting state tobacco companies in negotiating and signing production contracts with tobacco growers. In return, local governments collected 20% of the special agricultural product tax once the state tobacco companies had purchased the tobacco leaves from growers. As a result, such tax revenue comprised a major part of local government budgetary income in the tobacco-producing provinces. For example, Xiao Shi Qiao, a town in Yunnan, had total revenue of RMB 3.2 million in 2000, of which RMB 2.3 million came from the special agricultural tax on tobacco.

Economic contributions by the national tobacco monopoly translated into powerful political influence throughout the country. The political authority of the Chinese Communist Party (CCP) comes in part from its economic performance legitimacy—the credibility gained as a result of the rapid economic growth experienced in China since the CCP came to power.[11] As long as China's economy continues to grow, the CCP is likely to retain the mandate to govern. Consequently, the overriding goal of the CCP-run government has been to ensure that regulations, public health or otherwise, did not restrict economic development policy options or impede growth. In this context, public health has often been ignored and the Ministry of Health (MOH) in China is bureaucratically weak, often relying heavily on interagency cooperation to accomplish its policy goals. In regard to tobacco, government officials were also warned by tobacco industry interests that, in addition to the economic losses, tobacco control could be socially divisive and destabilizing for the country. Their argument was, and continues to be, rooted in the fear that the poor, who have become increasingly dispossessed of land, jobs, and human rights, could revolt if the price of tobacco, one of their few pleasures, was raised or if tobacco-related jobs were lost.

In addition to its economic influence, the CNTC's political power (especially in relation to the MOH) historically came from the institutional structures that linked it directly to policymaking. In 1982, the Chinese government undertook the modernization of the Chinese tobacco industry and gained greater control of tobacco production, marketing, imports, and exports.[12] China established both the CNTC, responsible for marketing, production, distribution, and sales of all tobacco products in China, and the STMA, which was responsible for regulating the CNTC and enforcing the domestic monopoly. In reality, the STMA controlled the CNTC in name only. They shared the same leadership, staff, and functions; therefore, one institution administered the national tobacco industry, performed the governmental functions of management and supervision, and operated a business with valuable commercial interests.[13]

The roots of China's domestic tobacco monopoly can be traced back to the activities of international tobacco firms at the turn of the last century. The American Tobacco Company began exporting cigarettes to China in the 1890s. When the American Tobacco Company broke up in 1911 as a result of anti-trust legislation in the United States, British American Tobacco (BAT) took over most of its Chinese operations. BAT dominated the domestic tobacco market in China throughout the first half of the twentieth century, never dropping below 50% market share until the communist party nationalized the company's Chinese holdings in 1952.[14] By the mid-1990s, the "modern" CNTC produced more than 1.7 trillion cigarettes per year, which were marketed under more than 900 brands. Many brands consisted of poor quality tobacco and were extremely cheap, selling for approximately 10 cents per pack.[15]

Transnational firms did not re-enter the Chinese market until the mid-1980s, when the government sought modest technical support to modernize its operations through joint ventures with a few multinationals. However, international efforts to break into the Chinese market remained largely unsuccessful. China imposed import quotas, high tariffs, and other trade barriers to keep foreign brands out. Consequently, foreign brands comprised less than 5% of the Chinese market in the late 1990s and were mainly available in large cities. The most common foreign brands were 555, made by BAT, and Mild Seven, made by Japan Tobacco International (JTI). Marlboro, Lucky Strike, Dunhill, and Benson and Hedges were also sought-after status symbols by cigarette smokers. One consequence of the government's policy toward foreign brands was the creation of a massive tobacco smuggling market. In the 1990s, 99% of foreign cigarettes sold in China were smuggled, resulting in more than $1.8 billion in lost government revenue annually. Evidence suggests that foreign tobacco companies, such as BAT, used illicit trade strategically to penetrate the Chinese market.[16]

The FCTC Process in China

Going into the FCTC process, China was largely concerned with ensuring that the treaty helped retain governmental control over its domestic tobacco market while using the process to enhance its reputation as a credible participant on the international scene. Both these factors might explain why China was among the 59 countries that pledged financial and political support for the FCTC at the fifty-second World Health Assembly in 1999. Despite this initial governmental support, the STMA was visibly antagonistic to the FCTC idea. During the FCTC public hearings in 1999, for example, the STMA argued, "The form, scope and scale of any tobacco controls must respect each country's different circumstances, and choices cannot interfere with national sovereignty."[17] Ironically, however, the most pressing issue on China's agenda at the start of the FCTC negotiations was ensuring that Taiwan did not use the process to gain international visibility and as an impetus to pursue its separatist policy. Going into INB1, Chinese negotiators were focused on assuring that Taiwan was not recognized as a party in the FCTC negotiations and the issue of Taiwan remained a core priority for the national leadership throughout the negotiations.

At the start of the negotiations, China established an inter-ministerial committee consisting of approximately a dozen (mainly governmental) agencies to set government-wide positions in relation to the negotiations. The National Development and Planning Commission (NDRC) led the committee. The NDRC is at heart an economic institution, with its core function being to analyze, formulate, and implement medium- and long-term national economic and social development strategies in the country. At the time of the FCTC negotiations, STMA was located within the NDRC. In addition to its representation through the NDRC, STMA was represented directly in the committee. Other agencies included the MOH, the State Economic and Trade Commission (SETC), and the Ministry of Foreign Affairs (MOFA).

Each of the institutions on the committee, including the STMA, sent representatives to one or more of the intergovernmental negotiating body (INB) sessions. The MOH, SETC, MOFA, STMA, and NDRC attended all six sessions. The membership of the Chinese delegation also included the highly esteemed Chinese Academy of Preventive Medicine (precursor to the China Center for Disease Control). The inclusion of STMA on the formal Chinese delegation and the designation of the NDRC representative as China's chief delegate received widespread criticism from other countries and NGOs given WHO's official policy banning participation of the tobacco industry. The Chinese government defended their action in the interest of "inclusiveness and openness."[18]

Negotiating Positions

Internal conflicts among the diverse Chinese delegation were evident from the start and manifested themselves through shifting positions taken by China during the negotiations. During INB1, for example, officials from the STMA found fault

TABLE 6

*Members of the Chinese Interministerial Committee on the FCTC Who Attended the Six
Negotiation Rounds of the WHO Framework Convention on Tobacco Control (FCTC)*

Institution	FCTC Negotiations					
	October 2000	April–May 2001	November 2001	March 2002	October 2002	February 2003
CAPM	1	1	1	1	1	1
GAOC	0	0	0	2	1	0
GAQSIQ	0	0	0	1	1	1
MOA	0	0	0	1	0	0
MOF	1	1	0	0	1	2
MOFA	2	2	2	2	2	2
MOH	3	5	4	4	4	3
Permanent Mission	0	1	1	1	1	1
SAIC	0	1	0	1	1	1
SAT	0	1	0	1	0	1
SDPC/NDRC	4	3	3	3	3	3
SETC	1	1	2	1	1	1
STMA	1	2	2	2	2	2
Total	13	18	15	20	18	18

CAPM, Chinese Academy of Preventive Medicine; GAOC, General Administration of Customs; GAQSIQ, General
Administration of Quality Supervision, Inspection and Quarantine; MOA, Ministry of Agriculture; MOFA, Ministry of
Foreign Affairs; NDRC, National Development and Reform Commission; SAIC, State Administration for Industry and
Commerce; SAT, State Administration of Taxation; SDPC, State Development and Planning Commission; SETC, State
Economic and Trade Commission; STMA, State Tobacco Monopoly Administration.

with the FCTC wording concerning "the devastating health, social, environmental and economic consequences of tobacco consumption," and they insisted that
the word "devastating" be removed. The frequent interventions by the STMA
representatives, as well as their claims that the MOH's support for tobacco control was a "betrayal of their country" and that at least one-tenth of the salaries of
MOH staff was paid through tobacco profits, gave the impression that China was
not serious about tobacco control or the FCTC.[19] It was evident at this point in
the process that the MOH did not have the leverage in the inter-ministerial bargaining process to counteract the influence of the STMA. The unwillingness of
the STMA to soften its opposition to certain textual proposals endured throughout the negotiations and continued to carry significant weight on the Chinese
delegation's deliberations and decision-making. Following INB1 in July 2001, for
example, the STMA formed a working group to study the treaty and proposed
counter-strategies for the chair's text. This working group continued to meet
through INB6.

    The influence of the STMA within the delegation and on official Chinese ne-
gotiating positions, however, took a sharp turn after INB1 due to an intervention
from China's top leadership. Before INB2, the State Council sent three explicit

instructions to the delegation. First, make all necessary efforts to ensure that the FCTC process results in a treaty. Second, don't argue over nuanced wording in the FCTC text. Third, continue to ensure that Taiwan does not gain visibility or succeed in pursuing its separatist policy.[20] The instructions sent a clear message to the STMA to quiet down and provided greater leverage to pro-tobacco control members of the delegation.

The appointment of the NDRC as the head of the delegation, so heavily criticized by outsiders at the time, has subsequently been viewed positively by Chinese tobacco control advocates. Xiong Bilin, an official in the Department of Industrial Development in the NDRC, was appointed to lead the delegation between INB3 and INB6. The Department of Industrial Development was in charge of long-term macroeconomic development and was not directly responsible for the STMA (then under the Department of Economic Development). Bilin signaled a shift in China's position toward a much stronger treaty, stating, "China devotedly supports WHO's efforts to control tobacco, appreciating the great influence of the FCTC, posing itself as a responsible power with completely cooperative attitude towards negotiation."[21] Bilin made clear the need to balance the different bureaucratic interests. On the one hand, he stressed the importance of the tobacco industry, saying that, "For a long time, Chinese economic development will depend on the tobacco industry to accumulate fiscal revenue and to partially solve the employment issue."[22] Conversely, he noted that as a responsible power, China should support tobacco control, and he took seriously the projected long-term costs of tobacco-related disease. Most importantly, as a representative of the NDRC, he had the power and will to neutralize the delegates representing the STMA (unlike the much weaker influence of MOH delegates), especially as the negotiations progressed. Consequently, China's position did not always reflect directly that of the Chinese tobacco industry as many had feared would be the case.

China's shift in approach toward the FCTC per the State Council's instructions had repercussions for the surrounding WHO Western Pacific region and benefited the FCTC process. Not wanting to seem less concerned about health than China, other resistors in the region, including Japan, were put under significant pressure to take comparable constructive positions toward the treaty. This pressure was particularly important in generating a Western Pacific regional consensus at the INBs, meaning that one country spoke on behalf of the entire region on those issues for which there was consensus. Not wanting to be seen as opposing the treaty, China agreed to participate in the regional consensus, which in the Western Pacific region was largely driven by small, and much more progressive (in relation to the FCTC), Pacific Island countries. China's involvement put pressure on Japan to also join the consensus. Consequently, throughout much of the negotiations, other FCTC-supportive countries often spoke on behalf of China and Japan (although both countries were clear that there were certain issues on which they had to speak independently). Notably, the United States and Germany, the two other strong treaty opponents, did not join in voluntary regional consensus groups.

In regard to specific textual proposals, China preferred a more generic FCTC, which would leave implementation guidelines to future protocols and domestic laws. China's strongest opposition during the negotiations focused on restrictions on marketing and advertising (article 13); health warnings, packaging, and labeling (article 11); and responsibilities and liabilities (article 19). Lack of Chinese support in these areas contributed to a less robust and more generic FCTC. During INB3, for example, the STMA representative argued that radical language used by the European Union, Canada, and other countries on warning labels was inappropriate for Chinese culture and that the use of pictorial warning labels would go against traditional Chinese culture and its domestic laws. During INB5, China received a Dirty Ashtray Award after the STMA representative made lengthy remarks seeking to water down the provisions that would allow people to use the convention to sue tobacco industries for compensation. Upset by the negative attention from NGOs, China joined the United States in seeking to deny NGOs access to the informal sessions during INB6. This action angered NGOs participating in the process and, as a result, China was awarded three additional Dirty Ashtray Awards from the Framework Convention Alliance (FCA) for its position toward civil society organizations. Chinese delegates took the issue up in the plenary discussions and have since testified that they were very upset about the impact of the awards on their efforts to establish a credible reputation during the negotiations.[23]

China also firmly opposed having price and tax measures in the treaty, although they were far from alone in this opposition. Many countries argued that tax policy should not be internationalized and that doing so would violate national sovereignty. However, unlike most other countries, China also strongly resisted restrictions on duty-free tobacco sales and was successful in softening related language in the final text. China joined the Big Four in challenging European countries' wishes to include strong language on liability as an "important means of rectifying damage caused by tobacco use"; the words "where necessary" were successfully added to article 19 to weaken its impact.

Although China's economic interests in defending its domestic industry often translated into opposition to strong commitments in the FCTC, occasionally these interests led to support for strong public health provisions. For example, during the second negotiating session, China was a vocal opponent of efforts led by the United States and Japan to include language prioritizing trade over tobacco control. Chinese officials were concerned that any language protecting trade over tobacco control would be used by transnational tobacco companies to pry open China's tobacco market.[24] Because of this opposition, China was awarded its one and only Orchid Award from the FCA (the only Orchid Award ever given to one of the Big Four).[25]

China was also a strong advocate for language concerning illicit trade—language that was eventually included in the final text. These positions on legal and illicit trade exemplify how China sought to use the FCTC to maintain absolute control of its domestic tobacco market. The ability of the FCTC to prevent and eliminate smuggling was also welcomed by the Chinese government as another mechanism for keeping foreign competitors out of its market.

Signature and Ratification

China signed the FCTC in November 2003 and ratified it in October 2005. The FCTC officially took effect in China on January 9, 2006. Whereas many international experts expressed surprise at Chinese ratification of the FCTC, domestic experts took ratification in stride as an anticipated outcome of a process heavily supported by the State Council and signed by the government. As is the case with Congress in the United States, after the government of China signs an international treaty, the People's Congress must ratify it. However, because China is a one-party country, the ratification process is typically more procedural than a forum for real debate. The government's participation in the development of, and stated commitment to, the FCTC in the past largely ensured an expeditious and procedural ratification. However, there was some delay and ongoing debate during ratification, with tobacco producers arguing that the treaty could complicate their business and that ratification should be delayed, and government officials arguing that ratification would not reduce government revenue.[26]

Post-FCTC Tobacco Control Environment in China

By ratifying the treaty, Chinese government officials were not necessarily signaling dedication to the goals of the FCTC or commitment to its implementation. China's history suggests that although China participates in global regulatory processes as a means of promoting its global power, global regulations are weakened or even neutralized through discretionary domestic enforcement.[27] FCTC implementation in the initial seven years after coming into effect in China largely reflected this tradition. Alternatively, some suggest that the Chinese government is taking a very long-term view in meeting its commitments, with the rationale that the "special situation of China" calls for caution in bringing about desired changes.

FCTC Implementation

In April 2007, the Chinese government created the Implementation Coordination Mechanism (ICM) to coordinate the implementation of the FCTC around the country. The ICM was initially led by the NDRC and included seven ministries: the MOH, MOFA, Ministry of Finance (MOF), the General Administration of Customs (GAOC), the State Administration for Industry and Commerce (SAIC), the General Administration of Quality Supervision, Inspection, and Quarantine (GAQSIQ), and the STMA (including CNTC).[28]

The structure of the ICM changed with 2008 Super Ministerial Reform, when the STMA was removed from under the control of the NDRC and integrated into the Ministry of Industry and Information Technology (MIIT). Unlike the long-range economic outlook of the NDRC, the MIIT is notorious for being market oriented, looking for short-term returns, and attempting to reduce government control in company management. Moreover, the STMA represents the only department in the MIIT responsible for tobacco-related issues and holds a seat on the ministry's influential party committee. The newly unrestrained STMA replaced the NDRC as the leader of the ICM and, therefore, the lead implementer of the FCTC in China.

The reorganized ICM with the STMA in the lead nearly guaranteed failure of effective implementation. The STMA's contempt for the FCTC continued well past the negotiation process. In 2006, the STMA produced a report written by a research group composed of more than 70 tobacco industry experts entitled *Counterproposal and Countermeasure Scheme Against the WHO FCTC.*[29] The STMA also translated the treaty document into Chinese, changing key words. For example, "should" was translated into "may," and "comprehensive" was translated into "extensive."[30]

There have been efforts to change the organization and hierarchy in the ICM. The MOH, for example, lobbied for its own leadership of the ICM, and in 2009, the MOH and the State Administration of Traditional Chinese Medicine (SATCM)

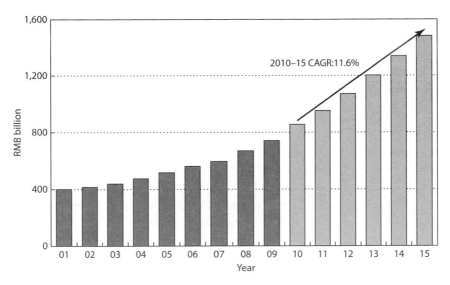

Figure 17. Compound annual growth rate (CAGR) in China's tobacco market. Data from Huabao, Credit Suisse Estimates

spearheaded the establishment of a National Healthcare System Leading Group (NHSLG) for FCTC implementation. In addition to the two initiators, the group included the Health Department of the General Logistics Department (GLD) of the Chinese People's Liberation Army (PLA) and the Logistics Department of the People's Armed Police Force (PAP).[31] To date, however, the STMA remains in charge of an ICM that is largely paralyzed by conflicts of interest.

Policy Change

For China to comply with the FCTC, a number of policy changes needed to occur after ratification. Among these were changes to youth access laws, advertising and promotion laws, and health warning labels on tobacco packages. However, instead of using the FCTC as the model, the STMA largely translated its *Counterproposal* report into national policy. Laws passed in 2007, for example, preventing the sale of tobacco products to minors failed to spell out punishments or say how they would be enforced. Similarly, the CNTC has taken advantage of loopholes in new advertising and promotion laws to continue marketing its products. The 2011 WHO Report on the Global Tobacco Epidemic gave China a score of five out of a possible ten points for compliance with direct bans on tobacco advertising, promotion, and sponsorship. Issues around price and tax also remained significant challenges.[32] In 2009, the Ministry of Finance raised taxes on tobacco products, but the STMA absorbed the increased cost to maintain the same retail price, therefore blunting whatever positive effect the tobacco tax increase may have had on reducing consumption.[33] Thus, the actual purchase price for most consumers went relatively unchanged. Opponents of the price increase used long-standing counterarguments, including stoking fear of social unrest if prices were raised for the poor.[34]

As foreshadowed during the negotiations, regulations on cigarette packaging and labeling became a hotly contested issue in China following FCTC entry into force. The STMA is directly responsible for mandating the content and style of health warnings on cigarette packages and remains staunchly against large, graphic warnings. China was awarded a Dirty Ashtray Award at the Conference of Parties in 2008 from the FCA after Chinese delegates argued that China refused to implement graphic health warnings on cigarette packages because "their placement next to beautiful Chinese landscapes currently on the packages would humiliate the Chinese public."[35] Other delegates viewed this interjection as ironic because of China's failure to recognize that these same cherished symbols were being used to sell death.

Revised STMA regulations on cigarette package labeling took effect in January 2009. The new warnings cover 30% of the packages (a requirement of the FCTC) but fail to describe the harm that tobacco use causes. The Chinese warnings read, "smoking harms your health" and "quitting smoking early helps reduce risk." The writing on one side is in tiny Chinese characters and in English on the other. Notably, there are approximately 85 million illiterate people in China and less than 30% of Chinese smokers can read English. In the end, there is very little difference between the pre- and post-FCTC health warning labels in China.[36]

On the five-year anniversary of the FCTC's entry into force in China, in January 2011, the Chinese Center for Disease Control released a critical report giving the Chinese government 37.3 out of 100 possible points in implementing the FCTC.[37] The report argued that tobacco was the top killer in China and criticized the tobacco industry's control of the policymaking process. The report, authored by public health expert Dr. Gonghuan Yang and Dr. Hu Angang, a respected academic economist, was widely covered by the Chinese media. Within two weeks, more than 900 related news articles had been published on the report.[38]

In February 2011, shortly after the report's release, the Chinese State Administration of Radio, Films, and Television ordered producers to limit the amount of smoking depicted on-screen and banned portrayals of minors under age 18 smoking or buying cigarettes. Characters in film and television productions also may not be shown smoking in public buildings or other places where smoking is banned.[39] In March 2011, the National People's Congress endorsed China's twelfth five-year plan, which mentioned tobacco control for the first time, calling for smoke-free public places.[40] In follow-up to the call for action in the five-year plan, the MOH issued a nationwide ban on smoking in hotels, restaurants, and other indoor public places. The regulation, however, excluded offices and government workplaces and lacked specific penalty provisions. The regulation relies on managers of public places to dissuade smokers without any applicable penalties for non-compliance. Enforceability is also problematic because enforcement rests with provincial and local governments. In China, the healthcare system is horizontally administered, meaning that those in charge of the local healthcare system are not responsible to the MOH but to local governments. Because many local governments look to tobacco for revenue, they are less motivated to enforce the regulations. There have also been no large-scale public awareness campaigns to promote the ban.

In 2013–2014 there was movement on the part of the National Health and Family Planning Commission (formerly the MOH) to draft a National Smoke-free Law that was placed on the State Council agenda. The draft was made available to international experts for review and comment, and there was clear support during the National People's Congress in March 2014 for a national law banning smoking in indoor public places by the end of 2014.[41] Notably, a circular from the Communist Party of China Central Committee and the State Council in December 2013 prohibited officials from smoking in public areas, including schools, hospitals, and sports venues, and on public transport.

Institutional barriers to tobacco control at the national level ensured by the STMA's leadership of the ICM have led many advocates to focus efforts on subnational and local governments where there has been some limited success. Smoke-free environments, for example, have been legislated in Beijing, Shanghai, Hangzhou, and Guangzhou, with Harbin being the first Chinese city to outlaw smoking in restaurants. However, progress at the local level has also proved to be extremely difficult, especially if there is tobacco growing in the region. Nanchang was set to implement a smoking ban in restaurants, bars, and other entertainment venues in 2013, for example, but the plan was delayed until 2015 after lawmakers blocked the law due to its tough wording.[42] In an analysis of media coverage of tobacco between 2000 and 2010, researchers found that national newspapers (funded by the national government) tended to be supportive of tobacco control efforts, whereas local newspapers (funded by local governments) were not.[43]

It should be noted that despite the lack of national policy progress, the number of motions for restrictive tobacco control and the amount of people making the motions have dramatically increased in the National People's Congress, the top lawmaking body. Tobacco control advocates have also sought to increase their influence on China's top leaders. Interestingly, in 2013 none of the nine members of the Politburo Standing Committee was a smoker, and only five members of the 25-member Politburo smoked (and they rarely smoked in public).[44] However, although there is little question that successful tobacco control in China will require support from China's top leaders, analysis of and influence on these individuals is extremely difficult. Information about top Chinese officials and their power interactions is notoriously secretive and highly unreliable. Unlike under Mao Zedong or Deng Xiaoping, however, today's leaders are thought to be more responsive to public opinion.[45]

Perhaps signaling some progress on the leadership's political will to rein in the tobacco industry, in December 2013, the China Party School, the main training institution of China's Communist Party, released a 200-page document detailing tobacco control recommendations, including the tightening of tobacco controls and curbing of the STMA's regulatory powers.[46] The document also suggests that the State Council establish a national tobacco control office or designate a specific health department to "take charge, supervising the control of tobacco in all processes from production to sales."[47] Such a step would essentially mean that the STMA would be relieved of its regulatory authority over tobacco. Although the report does not reflect government policy, it does suggest a major shift toward tobacco control in the party and indicates what might be coming in the near future.

Civil Society Engagement and Norm Change

Non-governmental activity around tobacco control has grown substantially in China since FCTC ratification. Notably, signing the FCTC legitimatized the domestic tobacco control movement, allowing NGOs to argue that they are not challenging government authorities, but rather working for the effective implementation of an approved treaty. In 2004, CASH changed its name to the Chinese Association on Tobacco Control (CATC), with approval from the Ministry of Civil Affairs. The CATC's official mandate is to unite local tobacco control organizations and voluntary workers of all sectors in participating and promoting national tobacco control activities and implementing the FCTC in China. Using the FCTC as a platform, the CATC has been able to successfully lobby the Ministry of Civil Affairs to cancel the Chinese Charity Award (a prestigious govern-

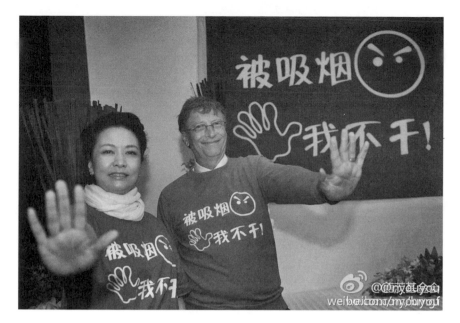

Figure 18. Bill Gates and Chinese First Lady Peng Liyuan, March 29, 2012. Bill Gates Foundation

ment award that recognizes outstanding corporate social responsibility) to six tobacco companies, lead a campaign to have the Shanghai World Expo organizing committee return RMB 200 million (approximately $30 million) it had received from the Shanghai Tobacco Group, and convince the eleventh National Games committee to return RMB 20 million ($3 million) in tobacco industry funding.[48] The CATC, in coalition with other domestic NGOs, also successfully pressured the Ministry of Civil Affairs to take back the Chinese Charity Award it had conferred on the CNTC.[49] In 2009, the CATC welcomed Peng Liyuan, China's then first lady, as their official anti-smoking ambassador.

The CATC, with extensive international support, is pushing for FCTC (and MPOWER) implementation in China. Since 2006, the CATC and other tobacco control groups in China have received generous financial support for tobacco control activities from the Bill and Melinda Gates Foundation and the Bloomberg Initiative to Reduce Tobacco Use. The Gates Foundation has provided approximately $24 million in grants, and the Bloomberg Initiative has dedicated even more. In addition, the China Medical Board has provided a domestic source of philanthropy in tobacco control. Initiatives carried out with this philanthropic funding include national anti-smoking campaigns on television and radio, educational programs with doctors, and a city-based project reaching 40 cities in 20 provinces and affecting more than 60 million people. Full-time positions focused on tobacco control in China have also been supported in domestic and international NGOs, as well as in the WHO China office.

The influx of external funding to Chinese tobacco control organizations was critical and its impact observable, especially in light of the meager national budget for tobacco control. In 2003, the Chinese government spent a total of $1 million on tobacco control, whereas cigarette sales generated $21 billion. During the past few years, this investment has grown to a measly RMB 9.6 million (approximately $3 million), or approximately 0.5% of the total budget for disease control and prevention. This budget helps employ only eight people in the Office of Tobacco Control, a standing office responsible for tobacco control affiliated with the MOH.[50] Since the launch of the Bloomberg Initiative in China, and with subsequent support from other donors, there has been a pronounced increase in professional trainings and technical and political meetings and conferences. Academic papers regarding tobacco issues in China have populated international peer-reviewed journals. Media coverage of the issue in the domestic and international press has increased markedly. There have, however, been some claims of external influence on domestic politics, and the CATC has been accused of serving its foreign sponsors instead of domestic public health interests.[51]

As has been the case in a number of countries, one of the most notable contributions from Bloomberg's financing was the execution of China's Global Adult Tobacco Survey (GATS), completed for the first time in 2010. GATS revealed both good and bad news for Chinese tobacco control advocates. In 2010, 52.9% of Chinese men were smokers. Although still dramatically high, this number represents a drop of approximately 10% in just over 10 years. The rate of smoking by Chinese women remains extremely low (2.4%). However, the GATS report showed that in contrast to other high-income countries, only 23% of adults in China were aware of the health risks of tobacco use, and an even smaller proportion of current users (16%) wished to quit. Ironically, slightly more adults (24%) believed that exposure to secondhand tobacco smoke causes heart disease and lung cancer in adults and lung illnesses in children. This lack of awareness extended to health professionals, 40% of whom continue to smoke. Nearly half of adults reported seeing anti-tobacco information on the television or radio in the past three months, although approximately 20% also noticed cigarette marketing, including on television (7.4%).[52]

Despite these sobering statistics, there is evidence to suggest that the Chinese

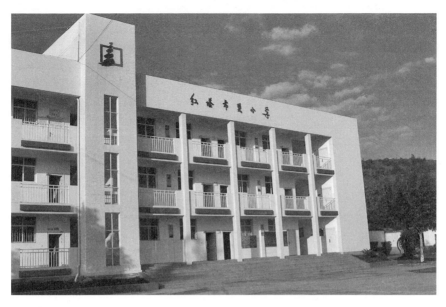

Figure 19. Tobacco-sponsored school in China: "Genius comes from hard work; tobacco can help you succeed." Theodore Curran

public is growing increasingly aware and supportive of tobacco control. In 2008, an online survey posted by the China Center for Disease Control generated 1.4 million affirmative responses in three weeks to China's implementation of the FCTC.[53] Particularly important on a symbolic and normative level, the Beijing Olympic Games in 2008 and the Shanghai World Expo in 2010 were both smoke-free events. China took advantage of both of these large international platforms to emphasize to the world its commitment to health.

There was perhaps no better example of China's past normative acceptance of the tobacco industry, and its rapidly changing position toward tobacco, than tobacco-sponsored schools. Just after China's ratification of the FCTC, the number of schools with tobacco-industry sponsorship increased rapidly. The most dramatic example was the primary school rebuilt after the Sichuan earthquake in 2010 with funds from a tobacco company. The school was initially named "Sichuan Tobacco Hope Primary School," and the school wall was inscribed with: "Talents are brewed by intelligence; tobacco helps you grow up and become accomplished."[54] In January 2014, however, the government banned smoking in schools and forbid schools from posting tobacco advertisements on campus, seeking sponsorship from cigarette brands, and selling cigarettes in school canteens.

Tobacco Industry Evolution

Ironically, despite areas of progress, the domestic Chinese tobacco industry has experienced an era of rapid growth since the FCTC entered in force in China. For example, 2009 was a landmark year for China's tobacco industry, with revenue (tax and profits) exceeding RMB 500 billion ($81.5 billion) while most other industries in the country witnessed significant drops in revenue. According to STMA director Jian Chengkang, the Chinese tobacco industry enjoyed approximately 19% annual growth between 2006 and 2010—the fastest growth rate of any industry in Chinese history.[55]

Much of this profitability is the result of ongoing modernization of the industry. This modernization has led to significant reduction in the number of brands, reduction in the number of small tobacco farmers (in an effort to improve leaf quality), and increased mechanization (leading to reductions in tobacco industry–related employment). Thus, despite its profitability and economic contributions amounting to more than $95 billion in tax revenue (5–8% of all government revenue), cigarette production is of declining importance to the overall economy, contributing less than 1% to the total value of industrial production.[56]

The strength of the industry, especially in light of an economic recession, has allowed the STMA leadership to play up the importance of the tobacco industry to China's economic development and play down commitments to the FCTC. This argument continues to fit perfectly with the CCP's development-first ideology and its performance-based legitimacy mindset.[57] There are reasons, however, to believe that the tobacco industry may not always have the direct line to policymaking power that it has had in the past. The STMA is occasionally referred to as the "last bastion" of the controlled economy.[58] Since the early 1990s, the central government has made the separation of government and enterprise functions a goal, and at each of China's legislative conferences since 1992, delegates have proposed the separation of the STMA and the CNTC. The 2008 Super Ministerial Reform was initially seen as an effort to free the STMA from the CNTC, allowing it to focus more on industry supervision.[59] However, thus far the institutional arrangements have failed to do this, and the STMA and the CNTC remain largely indistinguishable. Moreover, whereas rural agricultural taxes have been eliminated in recent years, there continues to be an exception for tobacco, making it one of the few crops through which rural governments can continue to control the market to raise revenue and finance themselves.

There is the possibility that economic cost arguments may have greater influence on policymakers in the future. Economic studies, largely funded by Bloomberg and Gates, have estimated that the economic costs of tobacco use in China range in the tens of billions of dollars.[60] Since market-oriented healthcare reform was ushered into China starting in the 1980s, the government has had little economic motivation to carry out tobacco control, because individuals are largely responsible for covering the direct healthcare costs from tobacco-related morbidity and mortality.[61] Recent changes resulting from healthcare reform efforts beginning in 2006 have shifted some of this responsibility to the government. Consequently, the calculations that the government must make in relation to the cost and benefits of tobacco control have shifted slightly. However, healthcare benefits remain quite low because one patient is only entitled to RMB 200 ($30) from the government under the New Rural Cooperative Medicare Scheme. Thus, smokers afflicted with tobacco-related diseases still must pay the lion's share of their medical costs for tobacco-induced diseases. China's healthcare reform has also not taken tobacco cessation into consideration; its national health insurance does not include the costs of nicotine replace therapy (e.g., gum, patches, lozenges) as recommended by WHO. The inclusion of indirect costs, such as workforce loss, may shift the government's calculations of the cost–benefit analysis of tobacco control.

Currently, China presents the global worst-case scenario for domestic FCTC implementation. Cultural norms, bureaucratic structures, and entrenched economic interests all continue to present complicated challenges to tobacco control. However, many advocates on the ground who have been working on tobacco control in China since the early 1990s point to remarkable changes that have taken place as a consequence of the FCTC. The simple fact that the Chinese government signed the FCTC means that it has legally acknowledged that smoking is harmful to public health and that the tobacco industry could have devastating consequences on the economy in the future. If nothing else, the FCTC provided the catalyst in China to expand the tobacco control debate beyond health experts to include the government, media, research institutions, and the public. Discussions surrounding FCTC implementation continue to engage government departments beyond those directly concerned with tobacco and health. Although the government has not committed significant financial resources to the tobacco control fight, international philanthropists, including Bloomberg and Gates, have stepped in to fill the gap.

China's few successes in tobacco control in the past ten years should not be underestimated. The adoption of laws that ban various forms of cigarette advertising, revised health warnings on cigarette packages, the passage of local legislation banning smoking in public places, progress towards a national smoke-free law, and the release of the China Party School's report on tobacco control are not trivial or inconsequential. Progress should be viewed in light of the relatively short history of tobacco control in China and the enormously challenging so-cio-political environment facing Chinese tobacco control advocates. As one advocate said, "While the meetings we are holding with policymakers don't seem to be having much impact, at least now we are having the meetings at all."[62] These meetings are growing more frequent and are involving higher-level party leadership. However, as long the tobacco industry is directly responsible for developing and enforcing tobacco control in the country, significant progress in reducing tobacco use and related disease and death will remain out of reach in China, and the global impact of the FCTC will be diminished.

CHAPTER NINE

Conclusion

A decade has passed since the entry into force of the Framework Convention on Tobacco Control—the world's first global health treaty. Although it is too soon to make any final statements on the treaty's long-term impact on tobacco-related morbidity and mortality, enough time has passed to evaluate how the process worked and to make initial judgments on the short-term value of the global process on domestic policy change. Close inspection of the process also offers insights beyond tobacco control, including into the role of the World Health Organization, the influence of non-state actors, and the future role of international legal regimes in the governance of global health.

One of WHO's primary rationales for institutionalizing tobacco control through the FCTC was the potential to intensify transnational communication and learning between policymakers and to instigate global policy diffusion. The evidence collected in this book indicates that the FCTC did fundamentally change the way tobacco control policy information was shared between countries and, consequently, accelerated the rate at which countries initiated policymaking processes and adopted new tobacco control measures. Individual interaction between tobacco control advocates was replaced by formalized transnational networking that took place regularly online and in person at international events affiliated with the FCTC process, including the intergovernmental negotiating bodies (INBs), regional intersessional negotiations, and technical workshops. These forums were used to frame the issues and communicate technical solutions to policymakers representing nearly every country in the world. Not only were these policymakers from diverse countries, but many came from non-health ministries, which further expanded the breadth of information sharing and knowledge generation during the process.

The impact of this communication on policy adoption is shown through quantitative analysis of the frequency and rate of tobacco control policy adoption before, during, and after the FCTC negotiations. A decade after its entry into force, more than 75% of parties to the treaty have strengthened existing legislation or adopted new policies. As observed globally, and detailed in the case studies in this book, the passage of stronger tobacco control policies has occurred in both FCTC-promoting countries and resistors. This evidence contradicts claims that legislative approaches to address global health issues take too long to implement and are too hard to enforce.[1]

The key element of any global "diffusion" process is the influence of communication and knowledge rather than coercion or legal obligation. Although the FCTC is binding, the overwhelming rise in policy change began well before the FCTC became international law. The case studies presented in this book also clearly document how technical information shared through the FCTC and the final treaty text influenced domestic knowledge of tobacco control. As a result, the primary motivation of policymakers in passing legislation was to improve public health as opposed to meeting international obligations. In all countries studied, the FCTC became an organizing principle during policy change discussions and a platform for domestic advocacy. Although Germany and China lag behind in legal implementation of the treaty obligations, advocates continue to push for full adoption and pressure policymakers to recognize the FCTC framework and align themselves with global norms.

The international governmental institutionalization of the FCTC provided the platform for diffusion to take place, but the process and impact was intensified by the participation of non-state actors—the global tobacco control community. The influence of the global tobacco control community was a recurrent theme throughout this book, starting with the foresight of longstanding members of the community (mainly medical doctors and public health professionals) who were able to frame the issue in a way that allowed for international institutionalization and regime formation in the first place. This foresight was followed by their ability to gain access to the top echelons of institutional leadership and to influence WHO decision making. The fact that the FCTC moved from a civil society–supported notion in 1994, largely considered implausible by WHO's legal leadership, to official WHO strategy four years later is a testament to the incredible political work done by members of the global tobacco control community in the intermediate years. However, the influence of civil society did not stop there. The impact of the global tobacco control community on the negotiations, through capacity building, technical assistance, and shaming, has been acknowledged by supporters and detractors and is formally recognized with the final treaty text.

There has been quite a bit written about the role and influence of transnational advocacy networks on issue creation, agenda setting, and global policy formation.[2] Fewer people have focused on how such networks extend their influence into domestic policy spheres. The descriptions of transnational partnerships and advocacy described in the case studies illustrate how transnational networks, such as the global tobacco control community, can extend their influence well beyond global discourses and be key actors in domestic policy processes. Although different domestic conditions and varying degrees of receptiveness for tobacco control require the development of contextualized advocacy and policy approaches for FCTC ratification and implementation, international financing and technical assistance has been pivotal at the national level.

Individual leadership in intergovernmental organizations, governments, and civil society was also indispensible throughout the FCTC process. Globally, the FCTC would not have been possible without the powerful leadership of WHO Director General Gro Harlem Brundtland. Her personal experience as a doctor defined the way in which she saw the world and reinforced her willingness to aggressively address tobacco use. However, it was her unique experience as prime minister of Norway that enabled her to build support for tobacco control at the highest levels of global financial institutions, the United Nations, and national governments, rather than relying on the support of health ministries.[3] She not only provided leadership publically, but she also led her WHO team through difficult political calculations (e.g., concerning trade in the final text) in assuring that the final treaty balanced strength with widespread acceptability.

Likewise, the existence of domestic tobacco control leaders with strong ties to the international network was instrumental in each case study. Notably, this is not just limited to the cases covered in this book, but is a consistent observation in countless other countries where one or two names are intimately linked to the tobacco control movement and have been so for years. For the most part, these individuals come from medical and public health backgrounds, but a common feature is their ability to successfully engage in policy formation and advocacy. As described in the previous case studies, national tobacco control advocates' access to the transnational network was strengthened during the FCTC process, and the technical assistance they received, as well as the final treaty instrument, bolstered their domestic influence and solidified their leadership.

Although individuals and non-governmental organizations undeniably sparked the emergence and influenced the outcome of the FCTC globally and domestically, at heart, the FCTC is a story of WHO leadership at a time when it was subject to harsh criticism. At the start of the FCTC process, WHO was thought to be mired in bureaucracy and lacking in global coherence and coordination across regions, control over priorities and funding, and the ability to represent all voices. Many of these criticisms continue to be leveled today, and WHO reform remains a popular, and never-ending, objective for the organization. In this context, it is important to acknowledge WHO's significant success in regard to the FCTC.

The FCTC is unique in international law because of the short time it took to negotiate and agree on a comprehensive and structured text, and because of its rapid entry into force and evident implementation in dozens of countries worldwide. This speed is reflective of the treaty's overwhelming buy-in and accepted legitimacy among WHO member states. The WHO secretariat, including its top leadership, headquarters staff, and regional offices, deserve recognition for this achievement.

The FCTC process typifies what WHO can uniquely offer in global health governance. WHO's organizational structure and formal administrative arrangements, like other intergovernmental organizations with lawmaking authority, allowed it to provide stable negotiating forums.[4] With substantial institutional support, nearly every single WHO member state participated in at least one of the INB sessions. The organizational structure of WHO, particularity the autonomy of its regional offices, has at times made it difficult to achieve unified goals. However, the FCTC process leveraged this regional autonomy to facilitate the negotiations, gain buy-in, and enhance equity. The active participation and influence of non-state actors counters prevailing arguments that WHO and other state-based institutions and processes devalue non-state participation.

Throughout the FCTC, WHO provided leadership on a critical emerging public health crisis and engineered governmental, non-governmental, and private partnerships to drive joint action. The FCTC process provided the forum through which evidence-based policy options were legitimatized, and it stimulated the generation, translation, and dissemination of knowledge. Above all, through the FCTC, WHO inspired its member states to set global norms and standards concerning state responsibilities in regard to tobacco control and to provide a framework through which to promote and monitor implementation.

However, despite this success, WHO's first international treaty faces significant challenges as it enters its second decade. There is palatable concern in the global tobacco control community that the best days of the FCTC may be behind it. Each of the trends highlighted—diffusion, civil society influence, and WHO leadership in tobacco control—are under threat. First, momentum regarding tobacco control has dissipated to some extent globally (notably having lasted far longer than may have been the case without the massive influx of funding from Bloomberg and Gates). Dips in momentum are typical in all efforts to sustain long-term global initiatives. Diffusion processes, by definition, reach a level of saturation, and a new innovation is required to catalyze new thinking and adoption processes. In the case of the FCTC, for example, ratification no longer drives global discourse, as the overwhelming majority of WHO member states are already party to the treaty, and approximately 70% have implemented its binding provisions. New transnational innovations are critically needed to sustain gains and for progress to continue. New approaches are also needed if the FCTC is to respond to the evolving global tobacco control environment.

The ability of the treaty to evolve might not seem like a significant barrier. As discussed in Chapter 3, framework conventions are, by definition, supposed to be good for rapidly changing conditions as they allow for iterative regime development through protocols. The fact is, however, that the development of protocols to the FCTC in the short term appears highly unlikely. The protocol process is at a complete standstill; the illicit trade protocol sits in limbo, and there is little political will to launch new negotiations relating to other elements of the FCTC. This is in part due to a general international movement away from treaty making. However, it also due to the significant lack of agreement within the global tobacco control community over how emerging issues in the global tobacco control environment should be handled. In regard to trade, for example, the global community is split between those who believe they must work within the existing frameworks of the global trade regime and those who believe that the tobacco control community must call for fundamental changes in the way tobacco and other health issues are addressed in existing and emergent agreements. In regard to e-cigarettes and other non-tobacco nicotine products, there is a divide between those who see such products as potentially beneficial for harm reduction (and even go so far as to endorse the products) and those who see the products as potentially dangerous and threatening to the hard-fought advances won against traditional tobacco use.

The FCTC story consistently demonstrates the power of the global tobacco control community to frame issues, set agendas, and drive policy change, and it also emphasizes the community's cohesion throughout the process. The global tobacco control community was repeatedly able to find universal consensus on issues and communicate this overwhelming agreement to policymakers with one voice. This cohesion was a key factor in ensuring the community's collective agency. For policymakers, the public health choices were clear. The dissolution of this unity weakens the community's message, its ability to set agendas, and consequently its influence in the process. In other words, it is impossible for policymakers to launch formal negotiations aimed at consolidating a global norm into binding law when no norm exists. The ability to reach consensus regarding the most pressing strategic decisions will only get more complicated as the network continues to diversify through broader alliances with activists in related fields, such as global development, global trade, or law enforcement. This difficulty has already been experienced in the case of the illicit trade protocol.

WHO leadership will be instrumental in keeping the global tobacco control community united and focused, and the role of WHO is critical in maintaining legitimacy, equity, and buy-in in global tobacco control governance. However, during the past decade, WHO's leadership in global tobacco control has been repeatedly challenged. The FCTC remains a "soft" international convention based largely on non-binding ideals, which deprives WHO of any substantial power to coerce its members to enforce FCTC policies. WHO has a been unable to withstand challenges to the FCTC from other international legal regimes, such as trade, and WHO's leadership has also been challenged by the influx of private funding and programming, including MPOWER. Adding to its struggle, WHO's funding crisis has resulted in reduced staff and led to the absorption of the Tobacco Free Initiative into a general non-communicable disease prevention department.

Challenges related to securing the funding needed to sustain momentum in FCTC implementation is not limited to WHO. Although private funding has been instrumental in implementing the FCTC to date, it has to some extent prevented the transnational tobacco community from aggressively seeking out innovative, sustainable funding solutions for domestic tobacco control programs. Economic austerity and competing priorities (even in the chronic, non-communicable disease realm) have resulted in funding cuts to public health in general, and tobacco control in particular. Even the Conference of Parties has been unable to agree on measures to secure the funds required to sustain FCTC implementation.

To retain some political attention and dedicated resources, a handful of members of the global tobacco control community continue to push for tobacco control to be recognized in the global sustainable development agenda, and they encourage their domestic counterparts to press for the inclusion of tobacco control in domestic development plans. To date, such efforts have experienced little success and will likely face ongoing challenges, in part because justifying tobacco control as a development concern complicates its historical rationale (economic security as opposed to public health or corporate accountability) and places tobacco control in direct competition with a broad range of other social and development priorities.

The FCTC's documented success as an instrument of policy diffusion, balanced with daunting challenges already realized and on the horizon, begs the question of whether similar international legal agreements should be used to address other global health issues in the future. The successful execution of the FCTC process, as well as the successful 2005 revision of the International Health Regulations, have resulted in calls for the elevation of WHO's lawmaking authority to a core function of the organization.[5] There have been numerous proposals for new global health treaties on issues such as alcohol and obesity, as well as calls for comprehensive treaties on global health.

There is no doubt that, to date, international health lawmaking is an underutilized tool. In areas with well-established, evidence-based regulatory approaches that protect public health, as was in place for tobacco control, the treaty-making process itself has proven an effective tool to advance global agreement and stimulate action. However, it is also essential to recognize that not all global health problems need to have an international legal solution. Significant success has also been experienced in other areas of global health during the past decade without the use of binding international law. In fact, the FCTC stands out in what was otherwise a decade defined by successful non-binding agreements and public–private partnerships regarding AIDS, malaria, tuberculosis, and vaccines.

Non-binding instruments may at times be more effective tools of global health governance than binding treaties, especially if the political will to initiate a binding process is lacking. Given their flexibility, non-binding instruments can facilitate compromise and cooperation among states with different goals and time horizons because states do not run risks to their international reputations or countermeasures if they break treaty commitments.[6] Moreover, consensus may be easier to achieve because non-binding standards do not involve formal legal commitments and the political sanctions they (may) entail. Notably, non-binding standards can be more easily updated and can more readily involve non-state actors, allowing them to be more responsive to the quickly changing world.

However, as we have repeatedly witnessed in the past, non-binding resolutions can lead to global inaction and domestic neglect. When dealing with aggressive corporations that negatively impact health, non-binding resolutions and self-regulation has been used to postpone effective global health solutions. The binding, legal nature of the FCTC forced states to pay attention and to extend the public health discussion well beyond ministries of health. Other issues that often fail to get the attention they deserve after numerous non-binding agreements and resolutions may very well benefit from legal solutions.

Nevertheless, even when legal solutions are considered, policymakers should think innovatively and strategically about the legal, substantive, and institutional options available rather than the narrow and heavily legalized treaty option used for tobacco. The 2001 United Nations General Assembly Special Session Declaration of Commitment on HIV/AIDS and the resulting Global AIDS Reporting Mechanism provide just one powerful alternative example. Unfortunately, efforts to replicate this process for non-communicable diseases fell short in terms of agreement on meaningful measures and resource allocation. Increasingly, there may be a need for mixed approaches that include both legal and non-binding measures to incentivize coordinated national and international action toward shared health goals in an increasingly complex global health governance environment.

Thanks to all those in WHO, governments, and civil society who worked to develop, adopt, ratify, and implement the FCTC, it is increasingly hard to find communities that are not protected by at least one effective tobacco control measure. Globally, tobacco is accepted as a health threat, and global norms dictate that governments of all incomes and forms must undertake specific evidence-based measures to prevent and control tobacco use among their citizens. As the FCTC enters its second decade, tobacco control advocates, WHO, and individual governments would be wise to remember lessons from the FCTC's first decade. These lessons include the power of international institutionalization to spark rapid and dramatic policy change domestically, the collective authority of unified non-state actors, the need for brave leadership to transform the status quo, the role of scientific evidence in supporting demands for change, and the need to hold transnational companies responsible for the global harm that emerges from unfettered corporate greed. Above all, they must remember that the global fight to prevent tobacco-related death and disease is far from over.

Ratification of the FCTC

Participant	Signature Date (day/month/year)	Ratification, Acceptance, Approval, Formal Confirmation, Accession, or Succession (day/month/year)	Entry into Force (day/month/year)
Afghanistan	29/06/2004	13/08/2010	11/11/2010
Albania	29/06/2004	26/04/2006	25/07/2006
Algeria	20/06/2003	30/06/2006	28/09/2006
Angola	29/06/2004	20/09/2007	19/12/2007
Antigua and Barbuda	28/06/2004	05/06/2006	03/09/2006
Argentina	25/09/2003		
Armenia		29/11/2004	27/02/2005
Australia	05/12/2003	27/10/2004	27/02/2005
Austria	28/08/2003	15/09/2005	14/12/2005
Azerbaijan		01/11/2005	30/01/2006
Bahamas	29/06/2004	03/11/2009	01/02/2010
Bahrain		20/03/2007	18/06/2007
Bangladesh	16/06/2003	14/06/2004	27/02/2005
Barbados	28/06/2004	03/11/2005	01/02/2006
Belarus	17/06/2004	08/09/2005	07/12/2005
Belgium	22/01/2004	01-11-2005	30/01/2006
Belize	26/09/2003	15/12/2005	15/03/2006
Benin	18/06/2004	03/11/2005	01/02/2006
Bhutan	09/12/2003	23/08/2004	27/02/2005
Bolivia (Plurinational State of)	27/02/2004	15/09/2005	14/12/2005
Bosnia and Herzegovina		10/07/2009	08/10/2009
Botswana	16/06/2003	31/01/2005	01/05/2005
Brazil	16/06/2003	03/11/2005	01/02/2006
Brunei Darussalam	03/06/2004	03/06/2004	27/02/2005
Bulgaria	22/12/2003	07/11/2005	05/02/2006
Burkina Faso	22/12/2003	31/07/2006	29/10/2006
Burundi	16/06/2003	22/11/2005	20/02/2006
Cambodia	25/05/2004	15/11/2005	13/02/2006
Cameroon	13/05/2004	03/02/2006	04/05/2006
Canada	15/07/2003	26/11/2004	27/02/2005
Cape Verde	17/02/2004	04/10/2005	02/01/2006
Central African Republic	29/12/2003	07/11/2005	05/02/2006
Chad	22/06/2004	30/01/2006	30/04/2006
Chile	25/09/2003	13/06/2005	11/09/2005
China	10/11/2003	11/10/2005	09/01/2006
Colombia		10/04/2008	09/07/2008
Comoros	27/02/2004	24/01/2006	24/04/2006
Congo	23/03/2004	06/02/2007	07/05/2007
Cook Islands	14/05/2004	14/05/2004	27/02/2005

Participant	Signature Date (day/month/year)	Ratification, Acceptance, Approval, Formal Confirmation, Accession, or Succession (day/month/year)	Entry into Force (day/month/year)
Costa Rica	03/07/2003	21/08/2008	19/11/2008
Côte d'Ivoire	24/07/2003	13/08/2010	11/11/2010
Croatia	02/06/2004	14/07/2008	12/10/2008
Cuba	29/06/2004		
Cyprus	24/05/2004	26/10/2005	24/01/2006
Czech Republic	16/06/2003	01/06/2012	30/08/2012
Democratic People's Republic of Korea	17/06/2003	27/04/2005	26/07/2005
Democratic Republic of the Congo	28/06/2004	28/10/2005	26/01/2006
Denmark	16/06/2003	16-12-2004	16/03/2005
Djibouti	13/05/2004	31/07/2005	29/10/2005
Dominica	29/06/2004	24/07/2006	22/10/2006
Ecuador	22/03/2004	25/07/2006	23/10/2006
Egypt	17/06/2003	25/02/2005	26/05/2005
El Salvador	18/03/2004		
Equatorial Guinea		17/09/2005	16/12/2005
Estonia	08/06/2004	27/07/2005	25/10/2005
Ethiopia	25/02/2004	25/03/2014	23/06/2014
European Union	16/06/2003	30/06/2005	28/09/2005
Fiji	03/10/2003	03/10/2003	27/02/2005
Finland	16/06/2003	24/01/2005	24/04/2005
France	16/06/2003	19/10/2004	27/02/2005
Gabon	22/08/2003	20/02/2009	21/05/2009
Gambia	16/06/2003	18/09/2007	17/12/2007
Georgia	20/02/2004	14/02/2006	15/05/2006
Germany	24/10/2003	16/12/2004	16/03/2005
Ghana	20/06/2003	29/11/2004	27/02/2005
Greece	16/06/2003	27/01/2006	27/04/2006
Grenada	29/06/2004	14/08/2007	12/11/2007
Guatemala	25/09/2003	16/11/2005	14/02/2006
Guinea	01/04/2004	07/11/2007	05/02/2008
Guinea-Bissau		07/11/2008	05/02/2009
Guyana		15/09/2005	14/12/2005
Haiti	23/07/2003		
Honduras	18/06/2004	16/02/2005	17/05/2005
Hungary	16/06/2003	07/04/2004	27/02/2005
Iceland	16/06/2003	14/06/2004	27/02/2005
India	10/09/2003	05/02/2004	27/02/2005
Iran (Islamic Republic of)	16/06/2003	06/11/2005	04/02/2006
Iraq	29/06/2004	17/03/2008	15/06/2008
Ireland	16/09/2003	07/11/2005	05/02/2006
Israel	20/06/2003	24/08/2005	22/11/2005
Italy	16/06/2003	02/07/2008	30/09/2008
Jamaica	24/09/2003	07/07/2005	05/10/2005
Japan	09/03/2004	08/06/2004	27/02/2005
Jordan	28/05/2004	19/08/2004	27/02/2005
Kazakhstan	21/06/2004	22/01/2007	22/04/2007
Kenya	25/06/2004	25/06/2004	27/02/2005
Kiribati	27/04/2004	15/09/2005	14/12/2005
Kuwait	16/06/2003	12/05/2006	10/08/2006
Kyrgyzstan	18/02/2004	25/05/2006	23/08/2006

Participant	Signature Date (day/month/year)	Ratification, Acceptance, Approval, Formal Confirmation, Accession, or Succession (day/month/year)	Entry into Force (day/month/year)
Lao People's Democratic Republic	29/06/2004	06/09/2006	05/12/2006
Latvia	10/05/2004	10/02/2005	11/05/2005
Lebanon	04/03/2004	07-12-2005	07/03/2006
Lesotho	23/06/2004	14/01/2005	14/04/2005
Liberia	25/06/2004	15/09/2009	14/12/2009
Libya	18/06/2004	07/06/2005	05/09/2005
Lithuania	22/09/2003	16/12/2004	16/03/2005
Luxembourg	16/06/2003	30/06/2005	28/09/2005
Macedonia (the former Yugoslav Republic of)		30/06/2006	28/09/2006
Madagascar	24/09/2003	22/09/2004	27/02/2005
Malaysia	23/09/2003	16/09/2005	15/12/2005
Maldives	17/05/2004	20/05/2004	27/02/2005
Mali	23/09/2003	19/10/2005	17/01/2006
Malta	16/06/2003	24/09/2003	27/02/2005
Marshall Islands	16/06/2003	08/12/2004	08/03/2005
Mauritania	24/06/2004	28/10/2005	26/01/2006
Mauritius	17/06/2003	17/05/2004	27/02/2005
Mexico	12/08/2003	28/05/2004	27/02/2005
Micronesia (Federated States of)	28/06/2004	18/03/2005	16/06/2005
Mongolia	16/06/2003	27/01/2004	27/02/2005
Montenegro		23/10/2006	21/01/2007
Morocco	16/04/2004		
Mozambique	18/06/2003		
Myanmar	23/10/2003	21/04/2004	27/02/2005
Namibia	29/01/2004	07/11/2005	05/02/2006
Nauru		29/06/2004	27/02/2005
Nepal	03/12/2003	07/11/2006	05/02/2007
Netherlands	16/06/2003	27/01/2005	27/04/2005
New Zealand	16/06/2003	27/01/2004	27/02/2005
Nicaragua	07/06/2004	09/04/2008	08/07/2008
Niger	28/06/2004	25/08/2005	23/11/2005
Nigeria	28/06/2004	20/10/2005	18/01/2006
Niue	18/06/2004	03/06/2005	01/09/2005
Norway	16/06/2003	16/06/2003	27/02/2005
Oman		09/03/2005	07/06/2005
Pakistan	18/05/2004	03/11/2004	27/02/2005
Palau	16/06/2003	12/02/2004	27/02/2005
Panama	26/09/2003	16/08/2004	27/02/2005
Papua New Guinea	22/06/2004	25/05/2006	23/08/2006
Paraguay	16/06/2003	26/09/2006	25/12/2006
Peru	21/04/2004	30/11/2004	28/02/2005
Philippines	23/09/2003	06/06/2005	04/09/2005
Poland	14/06/2004	15/09/2006	14/12/2006
Portugal	09/01/2004	08/11/2005	06/02/2006
Qatar	17/06/2003	23/07/2004	27/02/2005
Republic of Korea	21/07/2003	16/05/2005	14/08/2005
Republic of Moldova	29/06/2004	03/02/2009	04/05/2009
Romania	25/06/2004	27/01/2006	27/04/2006
Russian Federation		03/06/2008	01/09/2008

Participant	Signature Date (day/month/year)	Ratification, Acceptance, Approval, Formal Confirmation, Accession, or Succession (day/month/year)	Entry into Force (day/month/year)
Rwanda	02/06/2004	19/10/2005	17/01/2006
Saint Kitts and Nevis	29/06/2004	21/06/2011	19/09/2011
Saint Lucia	29/06/2004	07/11/2005	05/02/2006
Saint Vincent and the Grenadines	14/06/2004	29/10/2010	27/01/2011
Samoa	25/09/2003	03/11/2005	01/02/2006
San Marino	26/09/2003	07/07/2004	27/02/2005
São Tomé and Príncipe	18/06/2004	12/04/2006	11/07/2006
Saudi Arabia	24/06/2004	09/05/2005	07/08/2005
Senegal	19/06/2003	27/01/2005	27/04/2005
Serbia	28/06/2004	08/02/2006	09/05/2006
Seychelles	11/09/2003	12/11/2003	27/02/2005
Sierra Leone		22/05/2009	20/08/2009
Singapore	29/12/2003	14/05/2004	27/02/2005
Slovakia	19/12/2003	04/05/2004	27/02/2005
Slovenia	25/09/2003	15/03/2005	13/06/2005
Solomon Islands	18/06/2004	10/08/2004	27/02/2005
South Africa	16/06/2003	19/04/2005	18/07/2005
Spain	16/06/2003	11/01/2005	11/04/2005
Sri Lanka	23/09/2003	11/11/2003	27/02/2005
Sudan	10/06/2004	31/10/2005	29/01/2006
Suriname	24/06/2004	16/12/2008	16/03/2009
Swaziland	29/06/2004	13/01/2006	13/04/2006
Sweden	16/06/2003	07/07/2005	05/10/2005
Switzerland	25/06/2004		
Syrian Arab Republic	11/07/2003	22/11/2004	27/02/2005
Tajikistan		21/06/2013	19/09/2013
Thailand	20/06/2003	08/11/2004	27/02/2005
Timor-Leste	25/05/2004	22/12/2004	22/03/2005
Togo	12/05/2004	15/11/2005	13/02/2006
Tonga	25/09/2003	08/04/2005	07/07/2005
Trinidad and Tobago	27/08/2003	19/08/2004	27/02/2005
Tunisia	22/08/2003	07/06/2010	05/09/2010
Turkey	28/04/2004	31/12/2004	31/03/2005
Turkmenistan		13/05/2011	11/08/2011
Tuvalu	10/06/2004	26/09/2005	25/12/2005
Uganda	05/03/2004	20/06/2007	18/09/2007
Ukraine	25/06/2004	06/06/2006	04/09/2006
United Arab Emirates	24/06/2004	07/11/2005	05/02/2006
United Kingdom of Great Britain and Northern Ireland	16/06/2003	16/12/2004	16/03/2005
United Republic of Tanzania	27/01/2004	30/04/2007	29/07/2007
United States of America	10/05/2004		
Uruguay	19/06/2003	09/09/2004	27/02/2005
Uzbekistan		15/05/2012	13/08/2012
Vanuatu	22/04/2004	16/09/2005	15/12/2005
Venezuela (the Bolivarian Republic of)	22/09/2003	27/06/2006	25/09/2006
Vietnam	03/09/2003	17/12/2004	17/03/2005
Yemen	20/06/2003	22/02/2007	23/05/2007
Zambia		23/05/2008	21/08/2008

Chapter 1 · *A World Connected by Cigarettes and Disease*

1. Jordana, J., and D. Levi-Faur. "The Politics of Regulation in the Age of Governance." In J. Jordana and D. Levi-Faur, eds., *The Politics of Regulation: Institutions and Regulatory Reforms for the Age of Governance.* Cheltenham, UK: Edward Elgar Publishing, 2005.

2. van Waarden, F. "European Harmonization of National Regulatory Styles?" In J. A. E. Vervaele, ed., *Compliance and Enforcement of European Community Law.* The Hague: Kluwer Law, 1999.

3. Tews, K., P. E. R. O. Busch, and H. Jörgens. "The Diffusion of New Environmental Policy Instruments." *European Journal of Political Research* 42, no. 4 (2003): 569–600.

4. Hofstede, G. *Culture's Consequences: International Differences in Work-Related Values.* Vol. 5. Beverly Hills, CA: Sage Publications, 1980.

5. Zarsky, L. *Human Rights and the Environment: Conflicts and Norms in a Globalizing World.* Sterling, VA: Earthscan LLC, 2002.

6. Glasser, R. "We Are Not Immune—Influenza, SARS, and the Collapse of Public Health." *Harper's Magazine* (July 2004): 35–42.

7. Prescott, E. M. "SARS: A Warning." *Survival* 45, no. 3 (2003): 207–26.

8. Fidler, D. "Global Health Governance—Overview of the Role of International Law in Protecting and Promoting Global Public Health." World Health Organization, 2002.

9. Gostin, L. O. "A Framework Convention on Global Health: Health for All, Justice for All." *Journal of the American Medical Association* 307, no. 19 (May 16, 2012): 2087–92.

10. Lee, K., and Z. L. Brumme. "Operationalizing the One Health Approach: The Global Governance Challenges." *Health Policy Plan* 28, no. 7 (October 2013): 778–85.

11. World Health Organization. "10 Facts on Second-Hand Smoke," December 2009, http://www.who.int/features/factfiles/tobacco/en/.

12. World Health Organization. "Tobacco," May 2014, http://www.who.int/mediacentre/factsheets/fs339/en/.

13. Ibid.

14. Peto, R., and A. D. Lopez. "Future Worldwide Health Effects of Current Smoking Patterns." In C. Everett Koop, C. E. Pearson, and M. Rory Schwarz, eds., *Critical Issues in Global Health*. San Francisco: Jossey-Bass, 2001, 154–61.

15. Ruggie, J. G. "At Home Abroad, Abroad at Home: International Liberalisation and Domestic Stability in the New World Economy." *Millennium-Journal of International Studies* 24, no. 3 (1995): 507–26.

16. Commission on Global Governance. *Our Global Neighborhood*. Oxford: Oxford University Press, 1995.

17. Fidler, "Global Health Governance."

18. Gostin, "A Framework Convention on Global Health."

19. Lee and Brumme, "Operationalizing the One Health Approach."

20. Keohane, R. O. "Global Governance and Democratic Accountability." In D. Held and M. Koenig-Archibugi, eds., *Taming Globalization: Frontiers of Governance*. Cambridge, UK: Polity Press, 2003, 130–59.

21. Birnbaum, P. *States and Collective Action: The European Experience*. Cambridge, UK: Cambridge University Press, 1988.

22. Keohane, R. O., and H. V. Milner. *Internationalization and Domestic Politics*. New York: Cambridge University Press, 1996.

23. Lijphart, A. *Institutional Design in New Democracies: Eastern Europe and Latin America*. Boulder, CO: Westview Press, 1996.

24. Bennett, C. J. "What Is Policy Convergence and What Causes It?" *British Journal of Political Science* 21, no. 2 (1991): 215–33.

25. Jörgens, H. "Governance by Diffusion-Implementing Global Norms through Cross-National Imitation and Learning." In W. M. Lafferty, ed., *Governance for Sustainable Development: The Challenge of Adapting Form to Function*. Cheltenham, UK: Edward Elgar, 2004.

26. Tews, K., P.-O. Busch, and H. Jörgens. "The Diffusion of New Environmental Policy Instruments." *European Journal of Political Research* 42, no. 4 (2003): 569–600.

27. Jörgens, H. "The Diffusion of Environmental Policy Innovations—Findings from an International Workshop." *Environmental Politics* 10, no. 2 (2001): 122–7.

28. Kern, K., H. Jörgens, and M. Jänicke. "The Diffusion of Environmental Policy Innovations: A Contribution to the Globalisation of Environmental Policy." WZB Discussion Paper FS II 01-302 of the Social Science Research Center, Berlin, 2001.

29. Keohane and Milner, *Internationalization and Domestic Politics*.

30. Taylor, A. "The Framework Convention on Tobacco Control: The Power of the Process." Paper presented at the 11th World Conference on Tobacco or Health, Chicago, Illinois, August 2000.

31. Davies, D. "External Forces: Facing the Future." Paper presented at the TABEXPO Conference, Barcelona, Spain, November 26, 2003.

32. Levy, D. T., J. A. Ellis, D. Mays, and A.-T. Huang. "Smoking-Related Deaths Averted Due to Three Years of Policy Progress." *Bulletin of the World Health Organization* 91, no. 7 (2013): 509–18.

33. Taylor, A. L., T. Alfven, D. Hougendobler, S. Tanaka, and K. Buse. "Leveraging Non-binding Instruments for Global Health Governance: Reflections from the Global Aids Reporting Mechanism for WHO Reform." *Public Health* 128, no. 2 (2014): 151–60.

Chapter 2 · One Hundred Years in the Making

1. Brandt, A. M. *The Cigarette Century: The Rise, Fall, and Deadly Persistence of the Product That Defined America*. New York: Basic Books, 2007.

2. "Duke Homestead: Overview," last modified June 5, 2012, http://www.nchistoricsites.org/duke/main.htm.

3. Borio, G. "The Tobacco Timeline," last modified November 20, 2010, http://www.tobacco.org/resources/history/Tobacco_History.html.

4. Brandt, *The Cigarette Century*.

5. Fritschler, A. L., and J. M. Hoefler. *Smoking and Politics: Policymaking and the Federal Bureaucracy*. Englewood Cliffs, NJ: Prentice Hall, 1969.

6. Kiernann, V. G. *Tobacco: A History*. London: Hutchinson Radius, 1991.

7. US Department of Health and Human Services. *Preventing Tobacco Use among Young People: A Report of the Surgeon General*. Atlanta, GA: US Department of Health and Human Services, 1994.

8. Kiernann, *Tobacco*.

9. Lickint, F. "Tabak und Tabakrauch als Ätiologischer Faktor des Carcinoms." *Journal of Cancer Research and Clinical Oncology* 30, no. 1 (1930): 349–65.

10. Müller, F. H. "Tabakmissbrauch und Lungencarcinom." *Zeitschrift für Krebsforschung* 49 (1939): 57–85.

11. Jennings, H. S. *Biographical Memoir of Raymond Pearl, 1879–1940*. Washington, DC: National Academy of Sciences, 1943.

12. Doll, R., and H. Bradford. "Smoking and Carcinoma of the Lung: Preliminary Report." *British Medical Journal* 2 (1950): 739–48.

13. Levin, M., H. Goldstein, and G. Gerhardt. "Cancer and Tobacco Smoking." *Journal of the American Medical Association* 143 (1950): 336–8.

14. Wynder, G., and E. Graham. "Tobacco Smoking as a Possible Etiologic Factor in Bronchogenic Carcinoma." *Journal of the American Medical Association* 143 (1950): 329–36.

15. Wynder, E. L., E. A. Graham, and A. B. Croninger. "Experimental Production of Carcinoma with Cigarette Tar." *Cancer Research* 13, no. 12 (1953): 855–64.

16. Doll, R., and A. B. Hill. "The Mortality of Doctors in Relation to Their Smoking Habits: A Preliminary Report." *British Medical Journal* 1, no. 4877 (1954): 1451–5.

17. American Tobacco Companies. "A Frank Statement to Cigarette Smokers," 1954.

18. Henningfield, J. E., C. A. Rose, and M. Zeller. "Tobacco Industry Litigation Position on Addiction: Continued Dependence on Past Views." *Tobacco Control* 15 suppl. 4 (2006): 27–36.

19. Drope, J., and S. Chapman. "Tobacco Industry Efforts at Discrediting Scientific Knowledge of Environmental Tobacco Smoke: A Review of Internal Industry Documents." *Journal of Epidemiology and Community Health* 55, no. 8 (2000): 588–94.

20. Hurt, R. D., and C. R. Robertson. "Prying Open the Door to the Tobacco Industry's Secrets about Nicotine." *Journal of the American Medical Association* 280, no. 13 (1998): 1173–81.

21. Ong, E. K., and S. A. Glantz. "Constructing 'Sound Science' and 'Good Epidemiology': Tobacco, Lawyers, and Public Relations Firms." *American Journal of Public Health* 91, no. 11 (2000): 1749.

22. UK Royal College of Physicians. *Smoking and Health.* London: UK Royal College of Physicians, 1962.

23. US Public Health Service. "Smoking and Health: Report of the Advisory Committee to the Surgeon General of the Public Health Service." US Department of Health, Education, and Welfare, Public Health Service Publication, 1964.

24. "Cigarettes and Smoking" [Editorial]. *South African Medical Journal* 37, no. 39 (1963): 944–75.

25. Klein, N. *No Logo.* London: Flamingo, 2000.

26. Hirayama, T. "Non-smoking Wives of Heavy Smokers Have a Higher Risk of Lung Cancer: A Study from Japan." *British Medical Journal* 282, no. 6259 (1981): 183–5.

27. Trichopoulos, D., A. Kalandidi, L. Sparros, and B. MacMahon. "Lung Cancer and Passive Smoking." *International Journal of Cancer* 27, no. 1 (1981): 1–4.

28. US Department of Health and Human Services. *The Health Consequences of Involuntary Smoking: A Report of the Surgeon General.* Rockville, MD: US Department of Health and Human Services, 1986.

29. Drope and Chapman, "Tobacco Industry Efforts."

30. Barnoya, J., and S. Glantz. "Tobacco Industry Success in Preventing Regulation of Secondhand Smoke in Latin America: The 'Latin Project.'" *Tobacco Control* 11, no. 4 (2002): 305–14.

31. Pan American Health Organization. *Profits over People.* Washington, DC: Pan American Health Organization, 2002.

32. American Society of Heating, Refrigerating, and Air-Conditioning. *Environmental Tobacco Smoke Position Paper.* Atlanta, GA: American Society of Heating, Refrigerating, and Air-Conditioning, 2005.

33. Jacobs, R., H. F. Gale, T. C. Capehart, P. Zhang, and P. Jha. "The Supply-Side Effects of Tobacco Control Policies." In P. Jha and F. J. Chaloupka, eds., *Tobacco Control in Developing Countries.* Oxford: Oxford University Press, 2000, 311–42.

34. Mackay, J., and M. P. Eriksen. *The Tobacco Atlas.* Geneva: World Health Organization, 2002.

35. Crescenti, M. G. "The New Tobacco World." *Tobacco Journal International* 3, no. 51 (1998): 7.

36. Hammond, R. "Consolidation in the Tobacco Industry." *Tobacco Control* 7, no. 4 (1998): 426–8.

37. Ibid.

38. Shafey, O., S. Dolwick, and G. E. Guindon. *Tobacco Control Country Profiles.* Vol. 356. Atlanta, GA: American Cancer Society, 2003.

39. GYTS Collaborating Group. "Differences in Worldwide Tobacco Use by Gender." *Journal of School Health* 73, no. 6 (2003): 207–15.

40. Zatoński, W. *A Nation's Recovery.* Warsaw, Poland: Health Promotion Foundation, 2003.

41. Ibid.

42. Ibid.

43. National Association of the Tobacco Industry. "Tobacco Advertising Facts," 1998.

44. Mazur, J., B. Woynarowska, and A. Kowalewska. "Tobacco Smoking: Health of School-Aged Children in Poland." Faculty of Psychology, University of Warsaw, 2000.

45. Witold Zatoński, interview by author, November 2005.

46. Krzysztof Przewozniak, interview by author, 2005.

47. Malan, M., and R. Leaver. "Political Change in South Africa: New Tobacco Control and Public Health Policies." In J. de Beyer and L. W. Brigden, eds., *Tobacco Control Policy: Strategies, Successes, and Setbacks.* Vol. 628. Washington, DC: World Bank and Research for International Tobacco Control, 2003, 121–53.

48. de Beyer, J., and L. W. Brigden. *Tobacco Control Policy: Strategies, Successes, and Setbacks.* Vol. 628. Washington, DC: World Bank and Research for International Tobacco Control, 2003.

49. Frankel, G. "Thailand Resists U.S. Brand Assault." *Washington Post,* November 18, 1996.

50. Frankel, G. "U.S. Aided Cigarette Firms in Conquests Across Asia." *Washington Post,* November 17, 1996.

51. Rupert, J., and G. Frankel. "In Ex-Soviet Markets, U.S. Brands Took on Role of Capitalist Liberator." *Washington Post,* November 19, 1996.

52. GLOBALink homepage, accessed November 12, 2014, http://www.globalink.org.

53. Yach, D., and H. Wipfli. "A Century of Smoke." *Annals of Tropical Medicine and Parasitology* 100, no. 5-1 (2006): 465–79.

54. Mackay, J., and M. P. Eriksen. *The Tobacco Atlas.* Geneva: World Health Organization, 2002.

55. Zatoński, W. "Democracy and Health: Tobacco Control in Poland." In J. de Beyer, and L. W. Brigden, eds., *Tobacco Control Policy: Strategies, Successes, and Setbacks.* Washington, DC: World Bank and Research for International Tobacco Control, 2003.

56. Shafey, Dolwick, and Guindon, *Tobacco Control Country Profiles.*

57. Boyle, P., A. Onofrio, P. Maisonneuve, G. Severi, C. Robertson, M. Tubiana, and U. Veronesi. "Measuring Progress against Cancer in Europe: Has the 15% Decline Targeted for 2000 Come About?" *Annals of Oncology* 14, no. 8 (2003): 1312–25.

58. Yach, D., and D. Bettcher. "Globalisation of Tobacco Industry Influence and New Global Responses." *Tobacco Control* 9 (2000): 206–16.

59. Collin, J. "Think Global, Smoke Local: Transnational Tobacco Companies and Cognitive Globalisation." In K. Lee, ed., *Health Impacts of Globalisation: Towards Global Governance*. New York: Palgrave Macmillan, 2003, 61–86.

60. Yach and Bettcher, "Globalisation of Tobacco Industry Influence."

61. Crescenti, "The New Tobacco World."

62. Saloojee, Y., and E. Dagli. "Tobacco Industry Tactics for Resisting Public Policy on Health." *Bulletin of the World Health Organization* 78, no. 7 (2000): 902–10.

63. Pan American Health Organization, *Profits over People*.

64. World Health Organization. "Voices of Truth: Volume 1. Multinational Tobacco Industry Activity in the Middle East: A Review of Internal Industry Documents," 2007, http://www.who.int/tobacco/policy/en/vot1_en.pdf.

65. Ibid.

66. Ibid.

67. Zeltner, T., A. Kessler, A. Martiny, and F. Randera. *Tobacco Company Strategies to Undermine Tobacco Control Activities at the World Health Organization*. Geneva: World Health Organization, 2000.

68. Saloojee and Dagli, "Tobacco Industry Tactics."

69. Tobacco Free Initiative, World Health Organization. "WHO Resolutions," 2014, http://www.who.int/tobacco/framework/wha_eb/wha_resolutions/en/.

70. World Health Organization. *History of the WHO Framework Convention on Tobacco Control*. Geneva: World Health Organization, 2009.

71. Constitution of the World Health Organization, article 1, page 2, http://www.who.int/governance/eb/who_constitution_en.pdf.

72. Mihajlov, V. S. "International Health Law: Current Status and Future Prospects. Round Tale: Future of International Law." *International Digest of Health Legislation* 40 (2000): 9–16.

73. Ibid.

74. Roemer, R. *Legislative Action to Combat the World Tobacco Epidemic*. Geneva: World Health Organization, 1993.

75. Taylor, A. L. "Making the World Health Organization Work: A Legal Framework for Universal Access to the Conditions for Health." *American Journal of Law & Medicine* 18, no. 4 (1992): 301–46.

76. Roemer, R., A. Taylor, and J. Lariviere. "Origins of the WHO Framework Convention on Tobacco Control." *American Journal of Public Health* 95, no. 6 (2005): 936–8.

77. Mackay, J. "The Making of a Convention on Tobacco Control." *Bulletin of the World Health Organization* 81 (2003): 551.

78. Yach and Bettcher, "Globalisation of Tobacco Industry Influence."

79. WHO Resolution EB95.R9, An International Strategy for Tobacco Control, 95th session of the Executive Board, January 1995; WHA Resolution 48.11, 48th session, 12th plenary meeting, WHO Doc A48/1995/VR/12, May 12, 1995.

80. Ibid.

81. World Health Organization. *The Feasibility of an International Instrument for Tobacco Control*. Geneva: World Health Organization, WHO Executive Board Doc EB97/INF.Doc./4, 1995.

82. WHA Resolution 49.17, International Framework Convention for Tobacco Control, 49th session, 6th plenary meeting, May 25, 1996.

83. Roemer, Taylor, and Lariviere, "Origins of the WHO Framework Convention on Tobacco Control."

84. Reynolds, L. A., and E. M. Tansey, eds. *WHO Framework Convention on Tobacco Control.* Wellcome Witnesses to Twentieth Century Medicine, vol. 43. London: Queen Mary, University of London, 2012.

85. National Association of Attorneys General. Tobacco Master Settlement Agreement, 1998, http://publichealthlawcenter.org/sites/default/files/resources/master-settlement-agreement.pdf.

86. Vinocur, J. "North Sea Blowout Called 'Medium.'" *Pampa Daily News*, May 3, 1977.

87. Collin, J., K. Lee, and K. Bissell. "The Framework Convention on Tobacco Control: The Politics of Global Health Governance." *Third World Quarterly* 23, no. 2 (2002): 265–82.

88. United Nations Conference on Trade and Development. *Ad Hoc Inter-Agency Task Force on Tobacco Control—Report of the Secretary General.* New York: United Nations Conference on Trade and Development, 2000.

89. Ibid.

90. Jha, P., and F. J. Chaloupka. *Tobacco Control in Developing Countries.* Oxford: Oxford University Press, 2000; World Bank. *Curbing the Epidemic—Governments and the Economics of Tobacco Control: Development in Practice.* Washington, DC: World Bank, 1999.

91. Gallagher, P. J., ed. "Tobacco Regulation: The Convergence of Law, Medicine & Public Health—A Symposium in Celebration of the Inauguration of the William Mitchell College of Law's Center for Health Law & Policy." *William Mitchell Law Review* 25, no. 2 (1999).

92. World Health Organization. *Global Tobacco Control Law: Towards a WHO Framework Convention on Tobacco Control.* New Delhi: World Health Organization, 2000.

Chapter 3 · Those Who Want and Those Who Do Not . . . The FCTC Negotiations

1. United Nations. *Vienna Convention on the Law of Treaties.* Vienna: United Nations, 1969.

2. World Health Organization. "The Framework Convention on Tobacco Control: A Primer," 2003, http://whqlibdoc.who.int/hq/2003/WHO_NCD_TFI_99.8_Rev.7.pdf.

3. United Nations. "First Steps to a Safer Future: Introducing the United Nations Framework Convention on Climate Change," 2014, http://unfccc.int/essential_background/convention/items/6036.php.

4. United Nations. "Kyoto Protocol," 2014, http://unfccc.int/kyoto_protocol/items/2830.php.

5. Barker, J. C. "Mechanism to Create and Support Conventions, Treaties, and Other Reponses," 2004, http://www.eolss.net/eolsssamplechapters/c14/e1-44-01/e1-44 -01-txt-03.aspx.

6. World Health Organization. "Framework Convention on Tobacco Control: Technical Briefing Series," 1999, http://whqlibdoc.who.int/hq/1999/WHO_NCD _TFI_99.1.pdf.

7. Brundtland, G. H. *Seminar on Tobacco Industry Disclosures: Implications for Public Policy.* Geneva: World Health Organization, 1998, 2.

8. Taylor, A. L. "The Power of Process: The Impact of the WHO FCTC Negotiation Process on Global Public Health." Paper presented at the 11th World Conference on Tobacco or Health, August 19, 2000, Chicago, Illinois.

9. Tobacco Free Initiative, World Health Organization. *WHA52.18 Towards a WHO Framework Convention on Tobacco Control.* Geneva: World Health Organization, 1999.

10. World Health Organization. *History of the WHO Framework Convention on Tobacco Control.* Geneva: World Health Organization, 2009.

11. World Health Organization. *Proposed Draft Elements for a WHO Framework Convention on Tobacco Control: Provisional Texts with Comments of the Working Group, A/FCTC/INB1/2.* Geneva: World Health Organization, 2000.

12. Ibid.

13. Ibid.

14. Tobacco Free Initiative, World Health Organization. *WHA53.16 Framework Convention on Tobacco Control.* Geneva: World Health Organization, 2000.

15. Yach, D., and H. Wipfli. "A Century of Smoke." *Annals of Tropical Medicine and Parasitology* 100, no. 5–6 (2006): 465–79.

16. World Bank. *Curbing the Epidemic—Governments and the Economics of Tobacco Control. Development in Practice.* Washington, DC: World Bank, 1999, http:// documents.worldbank.org/curated/en/1999/05/437174/curbing-epidemic-govern ments-economics-tobacco-control.

17. Tobacco Free Initiative, World Health Organization. *Public Hearings on the WHO Framework Convention on Tobacco Control.* Geneva: World Health Organization, 2000.

18. Wipfli, H., D. Bettcher, C. Subramaniam, and A. Taylor. "Confronting the Tobacco Epidemic: Emerging Mechanisms of Global Governance." In M. McKee, P. Garner, and R. Stott, eds., *International Cooperation and Health.* Oxford: Oxford University Press, 2001. See also Framework Convention Alliance, "FCTC Public Hearings," 2001.

19. Framework Convention Alliance. "FCTC Public Hearings," 2001.

20. Wipfli et al., "Confronting the Tobacco Epidemic."

21. British American Tobacco. "British American Tobacco's Submission to the WHO's Framework Convention on Tobacco Control," accessed November 12, 2014, http://www.who.int/tobacco/framework/public_hearings/F0840080.pdf.

22. Assunta, M., and S. Chapman. "Health Treaty Dilution: A Case Study of Japan's Influence on the Language of the WHO Framework Convention on Tobacco Control." *Journal of Epidemiology and Community Health* 60, no. 9 (2006): 751–6.

23. Ibid.

24. Tobacco Free Initiative, World Health Organization. *Building Blocks for Tobacco Control: A Handbook*. Geneva: World Health Organization, 2004.

25. World Health Organization, *History of the WHO Framework Convention on Tobacco Control*.

26. Ibid.

27. Yach and Wipfli, "A Century of Smoke."

28. White, A. "Controlling Big Tobacco: The Winning Campaign for a Global Tobacco Control Treaty." *Multinational Monitor* 25, no. 1 (2004), http://multinational monitor.org/mm2004/04jan-feb/jan-feb04corp1.html.

29. Waxman, H. A. "The Future of the Global Tobacco Treaty Negotiations." *New England Journal of Medicine* 346, no. 12 (2002): 936–9. See also Hammond, R., and M. Assunta. "The Framework Convention on Tobacco Control: Promising Start, Uncertain Future." *Tobacco Control* 12, no. 3 (2003): 241–2; Gilmore, A. B., and J. Collin. "The World's First International Tobacco Control Treaty: Leading Nations May Thwart This Major Event." *British Medical Journal* 325, no. 7369 (2002): 846.

30. Waxman, "The Future of the Global Tobacco Treaty Negotiations."

31. Bates, C. "Developing Countries Take the Lean on the WHO Convention." *Tobacco Control* 10, no. 3 (2001): 209. See also Collin, J. "Tobacco Politics." *Development* 47, no. 2 (2004): 91–6.

32. Jacob, G. F. "Without Reservation." *Chicago Journal of International Law* 5, no. 1 (2004): 287–302.

33. Mamudu, H. M., and S. A. Glantz. "Civil Society and the Negotiation of the Framework Convention on Tobacco Control." *Global Public Health* 4, no. 2 (2009): 150–68.

34. Assunta and Chapman, "Health Treaty Dilution."

35. Wilkenfeld, J. P. "Saving the World from Big Tobacco: The Real Coalition of the Willing," 2005, http://www.gspia.pitt.edu/Portals/1/pdfs/Publications/Wilkenfeld .pdf. See also White, "Controlling Big Tobacco."

36. "Agents of Mass Destruction found in USA." *The Lancet* 361, no. 9369 (2003): 1575.

37. White, "Controlling Big Tobacco."

38. Yach and Wipfli, "A Century of Smoke."

39. World Health Assembly. "WHO Framework Convention on Tobacco Control," Article 4, Guiding Principle 7, WHA Resolution 56.1, May 21, 2003.

40. Jacob, "Without Reservation."

41. Zeltner, T., A. Kessler, A. Martiny, and F. Randera. *Tobacco Company Strategies to Undermine Tobacco Control Activities at the World Health Organization*. Geneva: World Health Organization, 2000. See also Ong, E. K., and S. A. Glantz. "Constructing 'Sound Science' and 'Good Epidemiology': Tobacco, Lawyers, and Public Relations Firms." *American Journal of Public Health* 91, no. 11 (2001): 1749.

42. Collin, J., K. Lee, and K. Bissell. "The Framework Convention on Tobacco Control: The Politics of Global Health Governance." *Third World Quarterly* 23, no. 2 (2002): 265–82.

43. World Health Organization, "History of the WHO Framework Convention on Tobacco Control."

44. Infact. "Treaty Trespassers: New Evidence of Escalating Tobacco Industry Activity to Derail the Framework Convention on Tobacco Control," February 2003.

45. Mamudu and Glantz, "Civil Society and the Negotiation of the Framework Convention on Tobacco Control."

46. Assunta and Chapman, "Health Treaty Dilution."

47. Mamudu, H. M., R. Hammond, and S. A. Glantz. "International Trade versus Public Health During the FCTC Negotiations, 1999–2003." *Tobacco Control* 20, no. 1 (2011): e3.

48. Ibid.

49. Ibid.

50. Intergovernmental Negotiating Body on the WHO Framework Convention on Tobacco Control. *New Chair's Text of a Framework Convention on Tobacco Control.* Geneva: World Health Organization, 2002, http://apps.who.int/gb/fctc/PDF/inb5/einb52.pdf.

51. Ibid.

52. United Nations. "Vienna Convention on the Law of Treaties."

53. Mamudu and Glantz, "Civil Society and the Negotiation of the Framework Convention on Tobacco Control."

54. Shapiro, I. S. "'Health versus Trade': Still Contentious." *Frame Convention Alliance Bulletin* 44 (2003), http://www.fctc.org/index.php/component/docman/cat_view/12-bulletins/21-inb6.

55. Panitchpakdi, S. "Director General Supachai Welcomes WHO Tobacco Agreement," *World Trade Organization News,* March 3, 2003, http://www.wto.org/english/news_e/news03_e/sp_who_tobacco_agr_3march03_e.htm.

56. Yach, D., H. Wipfli, R. Hammond, and S. Glantz. "Globalization and Tobacco." In I. Kawachi and S. Wamala, eds., *Globalization and Health.* New York: Oxford University Press, 2006.

57. Collin, J. "Global Health, Equity and the WHO Framework Convention on Tobacco Control." *Global Health Promotion* 17, no. 1 suppl (2010): 73–5.

58. Langley, A. "U.S. to Support World Tobacco-Control Treaty," *New York Times,* May 19, 2003, http://www.nytimes.com/2003/05/19/world/us-to-support-world-tobacco-control-treaty.html.

59. World Health Assembly. "WHO Framework Convention on Tobacco Control," WHA Resolution 56.1, May 21, 2003.

60. Framework Convention on Tobacco Control. "WHO Framework Convention on Tobacco Control," 2003: 1–42, http://www.who.int/fctc/text_download/en/.

61. Ibid.

62. Ibid.

63. Ibid.

64. World Health Organization, "History of the WHO Framework Convention on Tobacco Control."

65. Ibid.

66. Framework Convention Alliance. *Alliance Bulletin*, August 15, 2005, http:// www.fctc.org/publications/bulletins.

Chapter 4 · With Force: The First Decade of FCTC Implementation

1. World Health Assembly. "WHO Framework Convention on Tobacco Control," WHA Resolution 56.1, May 21, 2003.

2. World Health Organization. *History of the WHO Framework Convention on Tobacco Control.* Geneva: World Health Organization, 2009, http://whqlibdoc.who .int/publications/2009/9789241563925_eng.pdf.

3. World Health Organization. "Conference of the Parties to the WHO Framework Convention on Tobacco Control," 2014, http://www.who.int/fctc/cop/en/.

4. World Health Organization. "Global Progress Report on Implementation of the WHO Framework Convention on Tobacco Control," 2012, http://www.who.int /fctc/reporting/2012_global_progress_report_en.pdf.

5. World Health Organization. "Reporting Instrument," 2014, http://www.who .int/fctc/reporting/reporting_instrument/en/.

6. Ibid.

7. World Health Organization. "Report of the Secretariat on Its Activities," 2012, http://apps.who.int/gb/fctc/PDF/cop5/FCTC_COP5_4-en.pdf.

8. World Health Organization. "Parties' Reports," 2014, http://www.who.int/fctc /reporting/party_reports/en/.

9. World Health Organization. "WHO FCTC Implementation Database," 2014, http://www.who.int/fctc/reporting/implement_database/en/.

10. Plotnikova, E., S. E. Hill, and J. Collin. "The 'Diverse, Dynamic New World of Global Tobacco Control'? An Analysis of Participation in the Conference of the Parties to the WHO Framework Convention on Tobacco Control." *Tobacco Control.* Published online November 14, 2012. doi:10.1136/tobaccocontrol-2012-050849.

11. Ibid.

12. Thompson, F. "COP-3: In Praise of Smaller Countries." *Tobacco Control* 18, no. 2 (2009): 76.

13. Ibid.

14. World Health Organization. *Elaboration of Guidelines for Implementation of Article 5.3 of the Convention.* Durban, South Africa: Conference of the Parties to the WHO Framework Convention on Tobacco Control (Third Session), 2008.

15. Thompson, "COP-3."

16. Framework Convention Alliance. "Governments' Participation in Global Tobacco Control Efforts Threatened," 2012, http://www.fctc.org/index.php?option=com _content&view=article&id=809.

17. World Health Organization. *Relations with Nongovernmental Organizations: Report of the Standing Committee on Nongovernmental Organizations.* Geneva: World Health Organization, 2005.

18. Framework Convention Alliance. "2010 Tobacco Watch Report: Monitoring Countries' Performance on the Global Treaty." Published online November 12, 2010,

http://www.fctc.org/media-and-publications-20/reports/implementation-monitoring/443-tobacco-watch-monitoring-countries-performance-on-the-global-treaty.

19. World Health Organization. "Parties to the WHO Framework Convention on Tobacco Control." Published online November 27, 2013, http://www.who.int/fctc/signatories_parties/en/.

20. Mamudu, H. M., and S. A. Glantz. "Civil Society and the Negotiation of the Framework Convention on Tobacco Control." *Global Public Health* 4, no. 2 (2009): 150–68.

21. Harkin, T. "Harkin Urges President Bush to Reduce the Toll of Tobacco Use around the World." Published online July 19, 2005, http://www.harkin.senate.gov/press/release.cfm?i=240925.

22. American Lung Association. *Ratification of the Framework Convention on Tobacco Control (FCTC) Treaty.* Chicago: American Lung Association, 2014, http://www.lung.org/stop-smoking/tobacco-control-advocacy/federal/framework-convention-treaty.html.

23. US Congress. *Family Smoking Prevention and Tobacco Control Act*, 111th Congress, 2009–2010, H. R. 1256.

24. Xinhua. "Indonesia Ranked World's 3rd Largest in Smoking Habit." China.org.cn, published online January 25, 2011, http://www.china.org.cn/environment/2011-01/25/content_21812991.htm.

25. "Network Launches Road Map for Tobacco Control." *Jakarta Post,* published online June 26, 2013, http://www.thejakartapost.com/news/2013/06/26/network-launches-road-map-tobacco-control.html.

26. Faizal, E. B. "Ri Will Strive to Ratify Tobacco Control Convention." *Jakarta Post,* published online September 30, 2013, http://www.thejakartapost.com/news/2013/09/30/ri-will-strive-ratify-tobacco-control-convention-minister.html.

27. Framework Convention Alliance. "Argentina Passes Tobacco Control Law." Published online June 2, 2011, http://www.fctc.org/news-blog-list-view-of-all-214/general-news/549-argentina-passes-tobacco-control-law.

28. Mejia, R., V. Schoj, J. Barnoya, M. L. Flores, and E. J. Pérez-Stable. "Tobacco Industry Strategies to Obstruct the FCTC in Argentina." *CVD Prevention and Control* 3, no. 4 (2008): 173–9.

29. Golden Leaf Tobacco. "Still under Siege over Tobacco," 2013, http://goldenleaftobacco.net/index.php/media-library/news-a-events/75-still-under-siege-over-tobacco.

30. Ibid.

31. Johns, P. "COP-3: My Personal Impressions." *Tobacco Control* 18, no. 2 (2009): 76.

32. Ibid.

33. Framework Convention Alliance. "COP-2 Meeting Resources, 30 June–6 July 2007." Published online July 27, 2007, http://www.fctc.org/media-and-publications-20/meeting-resources/cop-2.

34. World Health Organization. *History of the WHO Framework Convention on Tobacco Control.*

35. World Health Organization. "About the Protocol to Eliminate Illicit Trade in Tobacco Products," 2014, http://www.who.int/fctc/protocol/about/en/.

36. Liberman, J. "The New WHO FCTC Protocol to Eliminate Illicit Trade in Tobacco Products–Challenges Ahead." *ASIL Insights* 16, no. 38 (2012), http://www.asil.org/insights/volume/16/issue/38/new-who-fctc-protocol-eliminate-illicit-trade-tobacco-products-%E2%80%93.

37. World Health Organization. "Ratification: Protocol to Eliminate Illicit Trade in Tobacco Products," 2014, http://www.who.int/fctc/protocol/ratification/en/.

38. Liberman, "The New WHO FCTC Protocol."

39. Ibid.

40. Report of the Convention Secretariat, Conference of the Parties to the WHO Framework Convention on Tobacco Control. Interim Performance Report for the 2012–2013 Workplan and Budget, Article 43, Doc. FCTC/COP/5/20, August 18, 2012.

41. Liberman, "The New WHO FCTC Protocol."

42. Conference of the Parties to the WHO Framework Convention on Tobacco Control. Applications for the Status of Observer to the Conference of the Parties, Note by the Convention Secretariat, Doc. FCTC/COP/5/3, August 9, 2012, http://apps.who.int/gb/fctc/PDF/cop5/FCTC_COP5_3-en.pdf.

43. Sollier, J., and R. Mangion. INTERPOL: A Partner in Curbing the Illicit Tobacco Trade, *Transnational Dispute Management* 5 (2012), http://www.transnational-dispute-management.com/article.asp?key=1876.

44. Myers, M. L. "Michael Bloomberg's Unprecedented Leadership in Global Tobacco Fight Will Save Millions of Lives," August 15, 2006, http://www.tobaccofreekids.org/press_releases/post/id_0936.

45. Bill and Melinda Gates Foundation. "Michael Bloomberg and Bill Gates Join to Combat Global Tobacco Epidemic," http://www.gatesfoundation.org/Media-Center/Press-Releases/2008/07/Michael-Bloomberg-and-Bill-Gates-Join-to-Combat-Global-Tobacco-Epidemic.

46. Ibid.

47. Institute for Global Tobacco Control, Johns Hopkins Bloomberg School of Public Health. "A Bloomberg Initiative Partner," accessed November 13, 2014, http://www.jhsph.edu/research/centers-and-institutes/institute-for-global-tobacco-control/about/designations/BI_partner.hmtl.

48. Bill and Melinda Gates Foundation, "Michael Bloomberg and Bill Gates."

49. Lopatto, E. "Mayor Bloomberg Donates $220 Million to Fight Smoking Abroad," March 22, 2012, http://www.bloomberg.com/news/2012-03-22/mayor-bloomberg-donates-220-million-to-fight-smoking-overseas.html.

50. Bill and Melinda Gates Foundation, "Michael Bloomberg and Bill Gates."

51. Johns Hopkins Bloomberg School of Public Health. "Leadership and Certificate Programs in Global Tobacco Control," accessed November 13, 2014, http://www.globaltobaccocontrolalumni.org/Leadership_Program/faq.html.

52. Centers for Disease Control and Prevention. "About GTSS," accessed November 13, 2014, http://www.cdc.gov/Tobacco/global/gtss/index.htm.

53. Stokes, C. "World's Largest Tobacco Use Study Possible by Grants to CDC Foundation." Published online August 17, 2012, http://www.cdcfoundation.org/blog -entry/worlds-largest-tobacco-use-study-possible-grants-cdc-foundation.

54. Ibid.

55. World Health Organization. "MPOWER: Advancing the WHO Framework Convention on Tobacco Control (WHO FCTC)," accessed November 13, 2014, http://www.who.int/cancer/prevention/tobacco_implementation/mpower/en/.

56. Velásquez, G. *Financial Implications of Emerging Challenges for the Implementation of the FCTC*. South Centre, Geneva: Harvard University, 2013.

57. Munzer, A. "The WHO FCTC: The Challenge of Implementation." *Lancet Respiratory Medicine* 1, no. 3 (2013): 182–4.

58. Bloomberg, M. "Accelerating the Worldwide Movement to Reduce Tobacco Use." Published online November 17, 2011, http://www.mikebloomberg.com/Bloom bergPhilanthropies2011TobaccoReport.pdf.

59. Campaign for Tobacco-Free Kids. "About the International Legal Consortium (ILC)," 2014, http://www.tobaccocontrollaws.org/learn-more/about-us/.

60. Allen, T. J. *Managing the Flow of Technology: Technology Transfer and the Dissemination of Technological Information within the R&D Organization*. Cambridge, MA: MIT Press, 1977.

61. World Health Organization. *WHO Report on the Global Tobacco Epidemic*. Luxembourg: World Health Organization, 2013.

62. Wipfli, H., and G. Huang. "Power of the Process: Evaluating the Impact of the Framework Convention on Tobacco Control Negotiations." *Health Policy* 100, no. 2–3 (2011): 107–15.

63. Sanders-Jackson, A. N., A. V. Song, H. Hiilamo, and S. A. Glantz. "Effect of the Framework Convention on Tobacco Control and Voluntary Industry Health Warning Labels on Passage of Mandated Cigarette Warning Labels from 1965 to 2012: Transition Probability and Event History Analyses." *American Journal of Public Health* 103, no. 11 (2013): 2041–7.

64. World Health Organization, *WHO Report on the Global Tobacco Epidemic*.

65. Ibid.

66. Levy, D. T., J. A. Ellis, D. Mays, and A.-T. Huang. "Smoking-Related Deaths Averted Due to Three Years of Policy Progress." *Bulletin of the World Health Organization* 91 (2013): 509–18, http://www.who.int/bulletin/volumes/91/7/12-113878/en/.

67. International Tobacco Control. "About ITC." last modified May 28, 2013, http://www.itcproject.org/about.

68. Fathelrahman, A., L. Li, R. Borland, H.-H. Yong, M. Omar, R. Awang, B. Sirirassamee, G. Fong, and D. Hammond. "Stronger Pack Warnings Predict Quitting More Than Weaker Ones: Finding from the ITC Malaysia and Thailand Surveys." *Tobacco Induced Diseases* 11, no. 1 (2013): 20.

69. International Tobacco Control. "Key Findings," last modified February 8, 2012, http://itc.media-doc.com/key_findings.

70. Giovino, G. A., S. A. Mirza, J. M. Samet, P. C. Gupta, M. J. Jarvis, N. Bhala, R. Peto, W. Zatonski, J. Hsia, J. Morton, K. M. Palipudi, S. Asma, and GATS Collabo-

rative Group. "Tobacco Use in 3 Billion Individuals from 16 Countries: An Analysis of Nationally Representative Cross-Sectional Household Surveys." *The Lancet* 380, no. 9842 (2012): 668–79.

71. Zellers, L. *Global Tobacco Control: What the U.S. Can Learn from Other Countries.* St. Paul, MN: Tobacco Control Legal Consortium, 2013, http://publichealthlaw center.org/sites/default/files/resources/tclc-synopsis-global-tobacco-control-zellers -2013_0.pdf. See also World Health Organization, "Health and Economic Impacts of Tobacco Use in Eurasia Working Group Countries," 2013.

72. World Health Organization. "Turkey's Transformation." *Bulletin of the World Health Organization* 90 (2012): 401–76, http://www.who.int/bulletin/volumes/90/6 /12-030612/en/.

73. Bloomberg, "Accelerating the Worldwide Movement."

74. Owusu-Dabo, E., A. McNeill, S. Lewis, A. Gilmore, and J. Britton. "Status of Implementation of Framework Convention on Tobacco Control (FCTC) in Ghana: A Qualitative Study." *BMC Public Health* 10, no. 1 (2010): 1.

75. Ibid.

76. Ibid.

77. Ibid.

78. Tumwine, J. "Implementation of the Framework Convention on Tobacco Control in Africa: Current Status of Legislation." *International Journal of Environmental Research and Public Health* 8, no. 11 (2011): 4312–31.

79. Framework Convention Alliance. "Monitoring Team Thwarts Tobacco Industry Interference in Uganda." Published online November 6, 2013, http://www.fctc .org/news-blog-list-view-of-all-214/industry-interference/1097-monitoring-team -thwarts-tobacco-industry-interference-in-uganda.

80. Ibid.

81. Ibid.

82. Ibid.

83. Gonzalez, M., L. W. Green, and S. A. Glantz. "Through Tobacco Industry Eyes: Civil Society and the FCTC Process from Philip Morris and British American Tobacco's Perspectives." *Tobacco Control* 21, no. 4 (2012): e1.

84. Wipfli, H. L. *Diffusion, Norms, and Governance: The Case of Tobacco Control.* Geneva: Université de Genève, 2007.

85. Yach, D. "The Origins, Development, Effects, and Future of the WHO Framework Convention on Tobacco Control: A Personal Perspective." *The Lancet* 383, no. 9930 (2014): 1771–9.

86. Ibid.

87. Stillman, F. A., and H. Wipfli. "New Century: Same Challenges." *British Journal of Cancer* 92 (2005): 1179–81.

88. Broughton, M. Chairman's speech from the British American Tobacco Annual General Meeting, London, April 21, 2004.

89. World Trade Organization, DS406, "United States—Measures Affecting the Production and Sale of Clove Cigarettes," April 24, 2012.

90. World Trade Organization, DS434, "Australia—Certain Measures Concern-

ing Trademarks and Other Plain Packaging Requirements Applicable to Tobacco Products and Packaging; Request for the Establishment of a Panel by Ukraine," August 17, 2012.

91. Philip Morris Asia Limited. "Notice of Arbitration: Australia/Hong Kong Agreement for the Promotion and Protection of Investments," November 21, 2011.

92. FTR Holdings SA (Switzerland), Philip Morris Products SA (Switzerland), and Abal Hermanos SA (Uruguay) v. Oriental Republic of Uruguay: Request for Arbitration. ICSID Case No. ARB/10/7, February 19, 2010.

93. For the European Free Trade Association court decision, see Philip Morris Norway v. the Norwegian State, represented by the Ministry of Health and Care Services. EFTA Case No. E-16/10, September 12, 2011.

94. South East Asia Tobacco Control Alliance. "Excluding Tobacco from Trade and Investment Agreements: Transpacific Partnership Agreement (TPPA)," 2013, http://seatca.org/dmdocuments/SEATCA%20Tobacco%20Carve%20out%20paper_FAQ.pdf.

95. Bollyky, T. "The Tobacco Problem in U.S. Trade." Council on Foreign Relations Expert Brief, September 5, 2013, http://www.cfr.org/trade/tobacco-problem -us-trade/p31346.

96. South East Asia Tobacco Control Alliance, "Excluding Tobacco from Trade and Investment Agreements."

97. Stillman and Wipfli, "New Century: Same Challenges."

98. Giovino et al., "Tobacco Use in 3 Billion Individuals from 16 Countries."

99. Stillman and Wipfli, "New Century: Same Challenges."

100. Heather, B. "Plain Packaging Legal Bill Could Be $8m." Published online September 3, 2013, http://www.stuff.co.nz/national/politics/8402739/Plain-packaging -legal-bill-could-be-8m.

Chapter 5 · The FCTC in Thailand: In Search of Solidarity

1. National Statistics Office, "National Health and Welfare Survey." Bangkok, Thailand, 1999.

2. Hamann, S. L., J. Mock, S. Hense, N. Charoenca, and N. Kungskulniti. "Building Tobacco Control Research in Thailand: Meeting the Need for Innovative Change in Asia." *Health Research Policy and Systems* 10 (2012): 2.

3. Vateesatokit, P. "Tailoring Tobacco Control Efforts to the Country: The Example of Thailand." In J. de Beyer and L. Waverley Brigden, eds., *Tobacco Control Policy: Strategies, Successes and Setbacks.* Washington, DC: World Bank and Research for International Tobacco Control (RITC), 2003.

4. Ibid.

5. Ibid.

6. P. Vateesatokit, interview by author, Bangkok, Thailand, December 2005.

7. Ibid.

8. TASCP. "One Million Children Will Eventually Die from Smoking," Bangkok, Thailand, 1988. See also Vateesatokit, "Tailoring Tobacco Control Efforts to the Country."

9. Tobacco Merchants Association. *US Cigarette Export Market Penetration in Thailand: A Multimillion Dollar Opportunity for US Leaf Producers*. Princeton, NJ: Tobacco Merchants Association, 1988.

10. Vateesatokit, "Tailoring Tobacco Control Efforts to the Country."

11. Ibid.

12. H. Chitanondh, interview by author, Bangkok, Thailand, December 2005.

13. Chitanondh, H. *Tobacco Use—An Update, 1991*. Bangkok, Thailand: National Committee for Control of Tobacco Use, Office for Tobacco Consumption Control, Ministry of Public Health, 1991.

14. H. Chitanondh, interview by author, Bangkok, Thailand, December 2005.

15. Chantornvong, S., and D. McCargo. "Political Economy of Tobacco Control in Thailand." *Tobacco Control* 10, no. 1 (2001): 48–54.

16. Vateesatokit, "Tailoring Tobacco Control Efforts to the Country."

17. Ibid.

18. Ibid.

19. Ibid.

20. P. Vateesatokit, interview by author, Bangkok, Thailand, December 2005.

21. Ibid.

22. Vateesatokit, "Tailoring Tobacco Control Efforts to the Country."

23. Chen, T. L., and W. M. Elaimy. *APACT: Development and Challenges in the Face of Adversity. Proceedings of the Third Asia-Pacific Conference on Tobacco or Health, June 1993, Omiya, Japan*. Tokyo, Japan: Asia-Pacific Association for the Control of Tobacco, 1994.

24. Vateesatokit, "Tailoring Tobacco Control Efforts to the Country."

25. General Agreement on Tariffs and Trade. *Decision: Thailand Restrictions on Importation of and Internal Taxes on Cigarettes, BISD 37s/200*. Geneva, Switzerland: World Health Organization, 1990.

26. Chitanondh, H. *The Passage of Tobacco Control Laws: Thai Davids versus Transnational Tobacco Goliaths*. Bangkok, Thailand: Thailand Health Promotion Institute, 2000.

27. Chantornvong and McCargo, "Political Economy of Tobacco Control in Thailand."

28. Ibid.

29. Vateesatokit, P., B. Hughes, and B. Rittiphakdee. "Thailand: Winning Battles, but the War's Far from Over." *Tobacco Control* 9 (2000): 122–7.

30. Chitanondh, *The Passage of Tobacco Control Laws*.

31. Ibid.

32. Ibid.

33. MacKenzie, R., J. Collin, K. Sriwongcharoen, and M. E. Muggli. "'If We Can Just Stall New Unfriendly Legislations, the Scoreboard Is Already in Our Favour': Transnational Tobacco Companies and Ingredients Disclosure in Thailand." *Tobacco Control* 13, suppl. 2 (2004): ii79–ii87.

34. Busai, S. "Disclosure of Cigarette Ingredients: Potential Domino Effect?" *Southeast Asian Journal of Tropical Medicine and Public Health* 25 (1994): 613–5.

35. Moreno, F. J. "PM Telex Urgent and Confidential from FJ Moreno to Dan Harris," Philip Morris, December 2, 1991, Bates No. 2023247396, http://legacy.library .ucsf.edu/tid/evu34e00.

36. Leung, A. "Thailand Ingredient Regulation," British American Tobacco, March 7, 1995, Bates No. 800162141, http://legacy.library.ucsf.edu/tid/izk42b00.

37. "The Secretariat of the Cabinet," accessed November 13, 2014, http://www .cabinet.thaigov.go.th/eng/aa_main11.htm.

38. Vateesatokit, "Tailoring Tobacco Control Efforts to the Country."

39. Trairatanobhas, V. "Re: Industry Meeting," February 23, 1993, Bates No. 304033687/3688, http://legacy.library.ucsf.edu/tid/xfp97a99.

40. Boyse, S. "Ingredients. British American Tobacco," April 15, 1994, Bates No. 503872506/2508, http://legacy.library.ucsf.edu/tid/kxi77a99.

41. Vateesatokit, "Tailoring Tobacco Control Efforts to the Country."

42. Riordan, M. " 'By Brand' Ingredients for Thailand" [BAT e-mail forwarded by Orm Porntipprapa to distribution], March 27, 1998, Bates No. 321112039/2040, http://legacy.library.ucsf.edu/tid/adh24a99.

43. Godby, P. "Thai Ingredient Law," August 18, 1999, Bates No. 321780987/0989, http://legacy.library.ucsf.edu/tid/zkh24a99.

44. Vateesatokit and Rittiphakdee, "Thailand: Winning Battles, but the War's Far from Over."

45. Ibid.

46. Chantornvong and McCargo, "Political Economy of Tobacco Control in Thailand."

47. World Health Organization. *Thailand Country Report on Tobacco Advertising and Promotion Bans*. Geneva, Switzerland: World Health Organization, 2003.

48. Ibid.

49. Ibid.

50. Campaign for Tobacco-Free Kids. "Country Case Studies: Thailand," 1999, http://global.tobaccofreekids.org/en/resources/by_country/thailand/.

51. Chantornvong and McCargo, "Political Economy of Tobacco Control in Thailand."

52. Ibid.

53. Ministry of Finance, Excise Department. "Annual Report: Cigarette Sales and Tax Revenue 1993," Bangkok, Thailand, 1994. See also National Statistics Office, "National Health and Welfare Survey."

54. Supawongse, C., and S. Buasai. *Evolution of Tobacco Consumption Control in Thailand* [in Thai]. Bangkok, Thailand: Department of Health, Ministry of Health, 1997.

55. Vateesatokit, "Tailoring Tobacco Control Efforts to the Country."

56. Ibid.

57. Ibid.

58. Lee, K., T. Pang, and Y. Tan. *Asia's Role in Governing Global Health*. New York: Taylor & Francis, 2013.

59. Shapiro, I. S. "Health versus Trade: Still Contentious." *Frame Convention Alliance Bulletin* 44, February 27, 2003, http://www.fctc.org/index.php/component /docman/cat_view/12-bulletins/21-inb6.

60. National Health Examination Survey Office. *Thailand National Health Examination Survey IV 2008–2009.* Bangkok: National Health Examination Survey Office, 2009.

61. Southeast Asia Tobacco Control Alliance. Southeast Asia Initiative on Tobacco Tax: Thailand, May 2013, http://tobaccotax.seatca.org/?page_id=105.

62. Macan-Markar, M. "HEALTH: Asia Tobacco Trade Fair Tests Thai Anti-smoking Policies." Inter Press Service, August 26, 2009, http://www.globalissues.org /news/2009/08/26/2620.

63. Vateesatokit, "Tailoring Tobacco Control Efforts to the Country."

64. Ibid.

65. Jantanamalaka, J. "Thailand Strengthening Alliances in South East Asia for Tobacco Control." Citizen News Service, March 2011, http://www.citizen-news.org /2009/03/thailand-strengthening-alliances-in.html.

66. Hamann, S. L., J. Mock, S. Hense, N. Charoenca, and N. Kungskulniti. "Building Tobacco Control Research in Thailand: Meeting the Need for Innovative Change in Asia." *Health Research Policy and Systems* 10 (2012): 3.

67. Ibid.

68. Vathesatogkit, P., T. Y. Lian, and B. Ritthiphakdee. *Health Promotion Fund: Sustainable Financing and Governance.* Bangkok, Thailand: Thai Health Promotion Foundation, 2013, http://seatca.org/?p=3032.

69. Southeast Asia Tobacco Control Alliance. *Malaysia's Proactive Way Forward in Anti-tobacco Proposal in Trade Agreement.* Bangkok: ASEAN Tobacco Control Resource Center, October 21, 2013, http://seatca.org/?p=3225.

Chapter 6 · The FCTC in Uruguay: Igniting a Global Leader

1. Seffrin, J. "Uruguay Football Team Should End Tobacco Industry Affiliation," Essential Action: Taking on the Tobacco Industry Across Borders, June 24, 2002, http://www.takingontobacco.org/media/seffrin0206.html.

2. Tobacco Free Initiative, World Health Organization. "Tobacco Free Sports—Play It Clean," World No Tobacco Day, 2002.

3. World Health Organization. "Kick-Off on World No Tobacco Day: The First Tobacco-Free World Cup," EURO Press Release, September 2002.

4. Ramos, A. *Economía del Control del Tabaco en Los Países del Mercosur y Estados Asociados: Uruguay.* Washington, DC: OPS, 2006.

5. Shafey, O., S. Dolwick, and G. E. Guindon. *Tobacco Control Country Profiles.* Vol. 356, Atlanta, GA: American Cancer Society, 2003.

6. Framework Convention Alliance for Tobacco Control. "FCA FCTC Monitor Report," 2007.

7. Shafey, Dolwick, and Guindon, *Tobacco Control Country Profiles.*

8. Global Youth Tobacco Survey Collaborative Group. "Youth: (Males and Females) Currently Use Any Tobacco Product, Grades 1–3 in Montevideo." *Uruguay-Montevideo GYTS Fact Sheet,* 2002.

9. Carbajales, A. R., and D. Curti. "[Fiscal Policy, Affordability and Cross Effects in the Demand for Tobacco Products: The Case of Uruguay]" [article in Spanish]. *Salud Pública de México* 52, suppl 2 (2010): S186–96.

10. Blanco-Marquizo, A. *Six Years That Changed Tobacco Control in Uruguay: Lessons Learned.* Washington, DC: PAHO, 2006.

11. Blanco-Marquizo, A. *Success Stories: Uruguay.* Global Smokefree Partnership, 2006.

12. Global Smokefree Partnership. "Smokefree Success Stories: Spotlight on Smokefree Countries." Campaign for Tobacco-Free Kids, accessed November 13, 2014, http://global.tobaccofreekids.org/files/pdfs/en/SF_success_uruguay_en.pdf.

13. Blanco-Marquizo, *Six Years That Changed Tobacco Control in Uruguay.*

14. Ibid.

15. Ibid.

16. Navas-Acien, A., A. Peruga, P. Breysse, A. Zavaleta, A. Blanco-Marquizo, R. Pitarque, M. Acuña, K. Jiménez-Reyes, V. L. Colombo, G. Gamarra, F. A. Stillman, and J. Samet. "Secondhand Tobacco Smoke in Public Places in Latin America, 2002–2003." *Journal of the American Medical Association* 291, no. 22 (2004): 2741–5.

17. The study is actually sited in the text of the decree: Uruguay Presidential Decree 268/05, 2005.

18. Blanco-Marquizo, *Six Years That Changed Tobacco Control in Uruguay.*

19. The International Tobacco Control Policy Evaluation Project. "ITC Uruguay National Report: Findings from the Wave 1 to 3 Surveys (2006–2011)," August 2012, http://www.itcproject.org/files/ITC_Uruguay_NR-Aug8-web-v2.pdf.

20. Blanco-Marquizo, *Six Years That Changed Tobacco Control in Uruguay.*

21. Ibid.

22. Ibid.

23. Ibid.

24. Tobacco Free Initiative, World Health Organization. "List of World No Tobacco Day Awardees—2005," http://www.who.int/tobacco/communications/events/wntd/2005/awards/en/index2.html.

25. Johns, P. "COP-3: My Personal Impressions." *Tobacco Control* 18, no. 2 (2009): 76.

26. Uruguay Presidential Decree 142/003, 2003.

27. Blanco-Marquizo, *Six Years That Changed Tobacco Control in Uruguay.*

28. Uruguay Presidential Decree 268/05, 2005.

29. Uruguay Presidential Decree 36/005, 2005.

30. Blanco-Marquizo, *Six Years That Changed Tobacco Control in Uruguay.*

31. Uruguay Presidential Decree 171/05, 2005.

32. Uruguay Ministry of Public Health homepage, accessed November 13, 2014, http://www.msp.gub.uy/.

33. Uruguay Presidential Decree 170/005, 2005.

34. Uruguay Presidential Decree 146/005, 2005.

35. Framework Convention Alliance for Tobacco Control. "Summary Report for Framework Convention Alliance." Presented at the International Workshop on Tobacco Control Legislation, Montevideo, Uruguay, August 15–16, 2005.

36. Uruguay Presidential Decree 36/005, 2005.

37. Tobacco Free Initiative, World Health Organization. "List of World No Tobacco Day Awardees—2006," http://www.who.int/tobacco/communications/events /wntd/2006/awards/en/.

38. Framework Convention Alliance for Tobacco Control. "FCA FCTC Monitor Report," 2007.

39. Ibid.

40. Blanco-Marquizo, *Success Stories: Uruguay*.

41. Framework Convention Alliance for Tobacco Control. "FCA FCTC Monitor Report," 2007.

42. Uruguay Ministry of Public Health. "Presidente Vazquez Lanzo Campaña: 'Un Millon De Gracias,'" February 20, 2006, http://www2.msp.gub.uy/uc_346_1.html.

43. Blanco-Marquizo, *Success Stories: Uruguay*.

44. Blanco-Marquizo, *Six Years That Changed Tobacco Control in Uruguay*.

45. The International Tobacco Control Policy Evaluation Project, "ITC Uruguay National Report."

46. Framework Convention Alliance for Tobacco Control. "FCA FCTC Monitor Report," 2007.

47. Blanco-Marquizo, *Six Years That Changed Tobacco Control in Uruguay*.

48. Framework Convention Alliance for Tobacco Control. "FCA FCTC Monitor Report," 2007.

49. Blanco-Marquizo, *Six Years That Changed Tobacco Control in Uruguay*.

50. The International Tobacco Control Policy Evaluation Project, "ITC Uruguay National Report."

51. Ibid.

52. Tobacco Free Initiative, World Health Organization. "MPOWER," accessed November 13, 2014, http://www.who.int/tobacco/mpower/en/.

53. Blanco-Marquizo, *Six Years That Changed Tobacco Control in Uruguay*.

54. The International Tobacco Control Policy Evaluation Project, "ITC Uruguay National Report."

55. Ibid.

56. Framework Convention Alliance for Tobacco Control. "FCA FCTC Monitor Report," 2007.

57. Weiler, T. "*Philip Morris vs. Uruguay*: An Analysis of Tobacco Control Measures in the Context of International Investment Law," Report No. 1 for Physicians for a Smoke Free Canada, July 28, 2010, http://italaw.com/documents/WeilerOpinion -PMI-Uruguay.pdf.

58. Ibid.

59. Hernandez, V. "Jose Mujica: The World's 'Poorest' President," *BBC Mundo*, November 14, 2012, http://www.bbc.co.uk/news/magazine-20243493.

60. Paolillo, C. "Part III: Uruguay vs. Philip Morris: Tobacco Giant Wages Legal Fight over South America's Toughest Smoking Controls," Center for Public Integrity, November 15, 2010, http://www.publicintegrity.org/2010/11/15/4036/part-iii-uruguay -vs-philip-morris.

61. Wilson, D. "Bloomberg Backs Uruguay's Anti-smoking Laws," *New York Times*, November 15, 2010, http://prescriptions.blogs.nytimes.com/2010/11/15 /bloomberg-backs-uruguays-anti-smoking-laws/?_r=2.

62. Abascal, W., E. Esteves, B. Goja, F. González Mora, A. Lorenzo, A. Sica, P. Triunfo, and J. E. Harris. "Tobacco Control Campaign in Uruguay: A Population-Based Trend Analysis." *The Lancet* 380, no. 9853 (2012): 1575–82.

Chapter 7 · The FCTC in Germany: An Island of Resistance

1. Watson, R. "United States and Germany Are Keen to See Tobacco Agreement Watered Down." *British Medical Journal* 326, no. 7398 (2003): 1055.

2. Grüning, T., H. Weishaar, J. Collin, and A. B. Gilmore. "Tobacco Industry Attempts to Influence and Use the German Government to Undermine the WHO Framework Convention on Tobacco Control." *Tobacco Control* (June 9, 2011), doi: 10.1136/tc.2010.042093.

3. Simpson, D. "Germany: How Did It Get Like This?" *Tobacco Control* 11, no. 4 (2002): 291–3.

4. Grüning et al., "Tobacco Industry Attempts to Influence."

5. Ibid.

6. Lehman, K. *Chemische und Toxikologische Studien über Tabak, Tabakrauch und das Tabakrauchen.* München, Germany: Oldenbourg, 1909.

7. Lickint, F. "Tabak und Tabakrauch als Ätiologischer Faktor des Carcinoms." *Journal of Cancer Research and Clinical Oncology* 30, no. 1 (1930): 349–65.

8. Frei, N. *Medizin und Gesundheitspolitik in der NS-Zeit.* München, Germany: Oldenbourg Verlag, 1991.

9. Proctor, R. N. *The Nazi War on Cancer.* Princeton, NJ: Princeton University Press, 2000.

10. Frei, *Medizin und Gesundheitspolitik in der NS-Zeit.*

11. Proctor, *The Nazi War on Cancer.*

12. Frankenberg, G. "Between Paternalism and Voluntarism: Tobacco Consumption and Tobacco Control in Germany." In E. A. Feldman and R. Bayer, eds., *Unfiltered: Conflicts over Tobacco Policy and Public Health.* Cambridge, MA: Harvard University Press, 2004, 161–89.

13. Hess, H. "The Other Prohibition: The Cigarette Crisis in Post-War Germany." *Crime, Law and Social Change* 25, no. 1 (1996): 43–61.

14. The VdC was dissolved after the departure of Philip Morris GmbH in May 2007 and re-established as Deutscher Zigarretenverband in March 2008 without Gallaher Deutschland GmbH (now part of Japan Tobacco International) and Philip Morris.

15. Bornhäuser, A., J. McCarthy, and S. A. Glantz. "German Tobacco Industry's

Successful Efforts to Maintain Scientific and Political Respectability to Prevent Regulation of Secondhand Smoke." *Tobacco Control* 15, no. 2 (2006): e1.

16. Glantz, S., J. Slade, L. A. Bero, P. Hanauer, and D. E. Barnes, eds. *The Cigarette Papers*. Berkeley: University of California, 1996.

17. Bornhäuser, McCarthy, and Glantz, "German Tobacco Industry's Successful Efforts."

18. Hirschhorn, N. "Shameful Science: Four Decades of the German Tobacco Industry's Hidden Research on Smoking and Health." *Tobacco Control* 9, no. 2 (2000): 242–8.

19. Ibid.

20. Ibid.

21. Grüning, T., A. B. Gilmore, and M. McKee. "Tobacco Industry Influence on Science and Scientists in Germany." *American Journal of Public Health* 96, no. 1 (2006): 20–32.

22. Ibid.

23. Dontenwill, W., H. J. Chevalier, H. P. Harke, U. Lafrenz, G. Reckzeh, B. Schneider. "Investigations on the Effects of Chronic Cigarette-smoke Inhalation in Syrian Golden Hamsters." *Journal of the National Cancer Institute* 51, no. 6 (1973): 1781–1832.

24. Ibid.

25. Bornhäuser, McCarthy, and Glantz, "German Tobacco Industry's Successful Efforts."

26. Hirschhorn, "Shameful Science."

27. Industry documents specifically identify approximately sixty scientists who received industry funding between 1975 and 1991 from the scientific department and committee of the VdC and individual transnational companies. However, this number is likely only a fraction of those who accepted funding from the broader network of tobacco industry–supported research institutes. See Grüning, Gilmore, and McKee, "Tobacco Industry Influence on Science and Scientists in Germany."

28. Berridge, V. "Why Have Attitudes to Industry Funding of Research Changed?" *Addiction* 92, no. 8 (1997): 965–8.

29. Grüning, Gilmore, and McKee, "Tobacco Industry Influence on Science and Scientists in Germany."

30. Colby, F. "Research Proposal to the German Cigarette Industry (Verband) on an Epidemiological Study on 'Passive Smoking' and Lung Cancer," June 16, 1982, http://legacy.library.ucsf.edu/tid/rnf35a00.

31. Körner, M. "Letter to E. Brückner, VdC, and Others," April 6, 1991.

32. Frankenberg, "Between Paternalism and Voluntarism."

33. Ibid.

34. Even today, the critical institutions for public health information in Germany, such as the Bundeszentrale für gesundheitliche Aufklärung, the central agency for health information of the federal government, are not adequately funded or staffed. See Frankenberg, "Between Paternalism and Voluntarism."

35. Simpson, "Germany: How Did It Get Like This?"

36. Ibid.

37. Frankenberg, "Between Paternalism and Voluntarism."

38. Deutscher Bundestag. "Auswirkungen des Zigarettenrauchens," Philip Morris, May 10, 1974, Bates No. 1000046931, http://legacy.library.ucsf.edu/tid/khj97eoo.

39. German Bundestag. "Gesundheitsschadliche Auswirkungen des Zigarettenrauchens" [Harmful Effects of Cigarette Smoking], May 5, 1975, http://legacy.library .ucsf.edu/tid/rri55doo.

40. Antje Huber, Federal Secretary for Youth, Family and Health. Speech at the 28th Scientific Congress of the Federal Association of Public Health Physicians, Inc., May 31, 1978, Bremerhaven, Germany.

41. Verband der Cigarettenindustrie. "Passive Smoking Presentation by the Verband der Cigarettenindustrie at the Occasion of the NMA'S Workshop in Washington, DC," September 20, 1983, http://legacy.library.ucsf.edu/tid/rsv32eoo.

42. Bornhäuser, McCarthy, and Glantz, "German Tobacco Industry's Successful Efforts."

43. Brückner, E. "Niederschrift über die Vorstandssitzung vom 900823," August 28, 1990, http://legacy.library.ucsf.edu/tid/fgr56eoo.

44. Krause, E. G. "IW-Gutachten Zu den Kosten Eines Nichtraucherschutz-Gesetzes Niveaulos Oder: Mit Welchen Methoden die Zigarettenindustrie, Gegen das Nichtraucherschutz-Gesetz Polemisiert." *Nichtraucher-Info* (1998): 12–13.

45. "Staatlich Verordneter Nichtraucherschutz Unerwünscht," *Lycos Nachrichten,* January 29, 1998.

46. Nichtraucher-Initiative Deutschland. "Pressemitteilung: Manipulierte Umfrageergebnisse zum Nichtraucherschutz-Gesetz [Press Release]." Munich: Nichtraucher-Initiative Deutschland, January 29, 1998.

47. Frankenberg, "Between Paternalism and Voluntarism."

48. Bornhäuser, McCarthy, and Glantz, "German Tobacco Industry's Successful Efforts."

49. Körner, "Letter to E. Brückner, VdC, and Others."

50. Bornhäuser, McCarthy, and Glantz, "German Tobacco Industry's Successful Efforts."

51. Frankenberg, "Between Paternalism and Voluntarism."

52. Ibid.

53. Ibid.

54. Ibid.

55. Ibid.

56. Ibid.

57. Ibid.

58. Ibid.

59. Ibid.

60. US Department of Health and Human Services. *Reducing the Health Consequences of Smoking: 25 Years of Progress. A Report of the Surgeon General.* Rockville, MD: US Department of Health and Human Services, Public Health Service, Centers

for Disease Control and Prevention, Center for Chronic Disease Prevention and Health Promotion, Office on Smoking and Health, 1989.

61. Frankenberg, "Between Paternalism and Voluntarism."

62. Ibid.

63. Bundesverfassungsgerichts. "BVerfGE 95:181," 1997.

64. Neuman, M., A. Bitton, and S. Glantz. "Tobacco Industry Strategies for Influencing European Community Tobacco Advertising Legislation." *The Lancet* 359, no. 9314 (2002): 1323.

65. Ibid.

66. Ibid.

67. Ibid.

68. Ibid.

69. Ibid.

70. Yach, D. "Global Dialogue for Health." Speech presented at Noncommunicable Diseases and Mental Health, World Health Organization, August 29–31, 2000, Hannover, Germany, http://www.who.int/tobacco/dy_speeches4/en/.

71. Fleck, F. "US and Germany Give Late Support to WHO Tobacco Accord." *British Medical Journal* 326, no. 7399 (2003): 1103.

72. Grüning et al., "Tobacco Industry Attempts to Influence."

73. Dirty Ashtray Award, *Alliance Bulletin* 45, February 28, 2003, http://www.fctc .org/publications/bulletins/doc_view/45-fca-bulletin-45-inb6.

74. M. Poetschke-Langer, interview by author, Washington, DC, July 15, 2006.

75. Duke, K. "World Cup Attacked for Failing to Ban Smoking." *British Medical Journal* 332, no. 7554 (2006): 1351.

76. "Germany Bows to Pressure and Stops Tobacco Advertising," EurActiv, June 15, 2006, http://www.euractiv.com/health/germany-bows-pressure-stops-tobacco -advertising/article-156134.

77. "Germany Gives in over EU Tobacco Advertising Ban," *Deutsche Welle*, June 14, 2006, http://dw.de/p/8cel.

78. Grüning, T., and A. Gilmore. "Germany: Tobacco Industry Still Dictates Policy." *Tobacco Control* 16, no. 1 (2007): 2.

79. A. Bornhäuser, interview by author, Baltimore, MD, February 2007.

80. Ibid.

81. Gilmore, A., and E. Nolte. "Germany: Tobacco Industry Makes Further Inroads." *Tobacco Control* 11, no. 4 (2002): 291.

82. Tuffs, A. "German Government under Attack for Anti-smoking Advertisements." *British Medical Journal* 327, no. 7411 (2003): 360.

83. Gilmore and Nolte, "Germany: Tobacco Industry Makes Further Inroads."

84. Simpson, "Germany: How Did It Get Like This?"

85. Caspers-Merk, M. "Continuing Influence of Tobacco Industry in Germany: Reply from the Drug Commissioner of the German Federal Government." *The Lancet* 360, no. 9341 (2002): 1255–6.

86. Hanewinkel, R., and B. Isensee. "One for Every 113 Inhabitants: Cigarette

Vending Machines in Germany." *International Journal of Epidemiology* 35, no. 4 (2006): 1104–5.

87. Ibid.

88. "Germany to Thwart Teenage Smokers with Credit Card Initiative," *Deutsche Welle,* May 12, 2006, http://dw.de/p/8Scx.

89. German Cancer Research Center, ed. *Tobacco Prevention in Germany—What Works?* From Science to Politics, Heidelberg, 2014, http://www.dkfz.de/de/tabakkon trolle/download/Publikationen/AdWfP/AdWfP_Tobacco_prevention_in_Germany _what_works.pdf.

90. Poetschke-Langer, M., and S. Schunk. "Germany: Tobacco Industry Paradise." *Tobacco Control* 10, no. 4 (2001): 300–3.

91. M. Poetschke-Langer, interview by author, Washington, DC, July 15, 2006.

92. M. Poetschke-Langer, interview by author, Heidelberg, Germany, September 15, 2004.

93. Ludwig, U. "Im Wurgegriff der Industrie." *Der Spiegel* 44 (May 5, 2005): 48.

94. Tuffs, A. "Public Health Scientists Accused of Soft Peddling the Dangers of Passive Smoking after Taking Grants from Tobacco Related Organisations." *British Medical Journal* 331, no. 7508 (2005): 70.

95. Poetschke-Langer and Schunk, "Germany: Tobacco Industry Paradise."

96. M. Poetschke-Langer, interview by author, Heidelberg, Germany, September 15, 2004.

97. Ibid.

98. Evers, M. "Das Ende der Toleranz." *Der Spiegel* 24 (2006): 64–76.

99. Ibid.

100. A. Bornhäuser, interview by author, Baltimore, MD, February 2007.

101. Duke, "World Cup Attacked for Failing to Ban Smoking."

102. Frankenberg, "Between Paternalism and Voluntarism."

103. Americans for Nonsmokers' Rights. "Germany," accessed October 27, 2014, http://www.no-smoke.org/goingsmokefree.php?id=577.

104. Ibid.

105. Frankenberg, "Between Paternalism and Voluntarism."

Chapter 8 · The FCTC in China: The "Responsible" Resistor

1. Callard, C. "Follow the Money: How the Billions of Dollars That Flow from Smokers in Poor Nations to Companies in Rich Nations Greatly Exceed Funding for Global Tobacco Control and What Might Be Done about It." *Tobacco Control* 19, no. 4 (2010): 285–90.

2. Hu, T.-w., Z. Mao, J. Shi, and W. Chen, *Tobacco Taxation and Its Potential Impact in China.* Paris: International Union Against Tuberculosis and Lung Disease, 2008; Ott, B., and R. Srinivasan. "Three in 10 Chinese Adults Smoke," *Gallup,* February 9, 2012, http://www.gallup.com/poll/152546/three-chinese-adults-smoke.aspx.

3. Mamudu, H. M., and S. A. Glantz. "Civil Society and the Negotiation of the Framework Convention on Tobacco Control." *Global Public Health* 4, no. 2 (2009): 160.

4. Malone, R. E. "China's Chances, China's Choices in Global Tobacco Control." *Tobacco Control* 19, no. 1 (2010): 1–2.

5. Yang, G., L. Fan, J. Tan, G. Qi, Y. Zhang, J. M. Samet, C. E. Taylor, K. Becker, and J. Xu. "Smoking in China: Findings of the 1996 National Prevalence Survey." *Journal of the American Medical Association* 282, no. 13 (1999): 1247–53.

6. Hu et al., "Tobacco Taxation and Its Potential Impact in China."

7. "Conversation with Judith Mackay." *Addiction* 108 (2013): 1897–1904.

8. Malone, "China's Chances, China's Choices."

9. Juan, S. "Report: Smoking Industry Harming Economic Health," *China Daily*, July 1, 2011, http://www.chinadaily.com.cn/china/2011-01/07/content_11805846.htm.

10. Food and Agriculture Organization of the United Nations. *Issues in the Global Tobacco Economy: Selected Case Studies*. Rome: Food and Agriculture Organization of the United Nations, 2003.

11. Jin, J. "FCTC and China's Politics of Tobacco Control." Presented at the 4th GLF Annual Colloquium, May 15, 2012, Princeton University, http://www.princeton.edu/~pcglobal/conferences/GLF/jin.pdf.

12. Ibid.

13. Zhang, H. " 'Yan Cao Di Guo' Xin Zhang Men" [The New Leader of Tobacco Empire], *Liaowang Dongfang Zhoukan (Guangzhou: Oriental Outlook)*, 2013, http://wen.oeeee.com/a/20130603/1063593.html.

14. Lee, K., A. B. Gilmore, and J. Collin. "Breaking and Re-entering: British American Tobacco in China 1979–2000." *Tobacco Control* 13, suppl 2 (2004): ii88–95.

15. There were, however, high-quality national brands, such as special edition releases of Panda cigarettes that could sell for $50 per pack.

16. Collin, J., E. LeGresley, R. MacKenzie, S. Lawrence, and K. Lee. "Complicity in Contraband: British American Tobacco and Cigarette Smuggling in Asia." *Tobacco Control* 13, suppl. 2 (2004): ii104–11. See also Lee, K., and J. Collin. " 'Key to the Future': British American Tobacco and Cigarette Smuggling in China." *PLoS Med* 3, no. 7 (2006): e228.

17. World Health Organization. *Global Tobacco Treaty Hearings: Public Hearings on the World Health Organization's (WHO) Proposed Global Treaty Framework Convention on Tobacco Control (FCTC)*. Geneva: World Health Organization, 2000: 1.

18. Lee, K., and Z. L. Brumme. "Operationalizing the One Health Approach: The Global Governance Challenges." *Health Policy Plan* 28, no. 7 (2013): 778–85.

19. Gao, F. "Gei 'Kong Yan Jiushi Maiguo' Lun Piao Lengshui [Criticism on the Opinion That Tobacco Control Was a Betrayal of the Country]." *CPC News* (2012): 1, http://cpc.people.com.cn/pinglun/GB/241220/18140339.html.

20. Cao, L. "Zhuanfang Guojia Kongyanban Zhuren Yang Gonghuan" [Interview with Yang Gonghuan, Director of China National Tobacco Control Office]. *Lifeweek*, 2010.

21. "An Interview with Xiong Bilin, Head of China's Delegation to FCTC Negotiation," *Tobacco China* 2010, http://www.tobaccochina.com/people/interview/wu/20037/200372110472_164827.shtml.

22. Huang, Y. "China's Position in Negotiating the Framework Convention on

Tobacco Control and the Revised International Health Regulations." *Public Health* 128, no. 2 (2014): 161–6.

23. Campaign for Tobacco-Free Kids. "Statement of the STMA Office On 'Dirty Ashtray Award,'" March 17, 2014, http://tobaccofreekids.meihua.info/InfoItemView .aspx?itemid=dfdc816c-1c3c-4ea6-a45d-a4dfb6b6c66f&u=Martin_miao&e=em.

24. Jin, "FCTC and China's Politics of Tobacco Control."

25. Mamudu and Glantz, "Civil Society and the Negotiation of the FCTC."

26. Jin, J. "Why FCTC Policies Haven't Been Transferred in China: Domestic Dynamics and Tobacco Governance." *Journal of Health Politics, Policy and Law,* March 6, 2014, doi:10.1215/03616878-2682630.

27. Jin, "FCTC and China's Politics of Tobacco Control."

28. Yang, G., and A. Hu. *Kongyan Yu Zhongguo Weilai: Zhongwai Zhuanjia Zhongguo Yancao Shiyong Yu Yancao Kongzhi Lianhe Pinggu Baogao [Tobacco Control and China's Future: Chinese and Foreign Experts Joint Evaluation Report on China's Tobacco Consumption and Tobacco Control].* Beijing: Jingji Ribao Chubanshe, 2011.

29. Zhou, R., and Y. Cheng. *Counterproposal and Countermeasure Scheme against WHO FCTC.* Beijing, China: Economic Science Publishing House, 2006.

30. Jin, "FCTC and China's Politics of Tobacco Control."

31. Fan, S. "Ministry of Health, State Administration of Traditional Chinese Medicine (SATCM), the Health Department of the General Logistics Department (GLD) of the Chinese People's Liberation Army (PLA) and the Logistics Department of the People's Armed Police Force (PAP) Decide to Systematically Ban Smoking in the National Healthcare System with Effect from 2011." *Journal of Preventive Medicine of Chinese People's Liberation Army* 28, no. 2 (2010): 1, http://d.wanfangdata.com.cn /periodical_jfjyfyxzz201002033.aspx.

32. World Health Organization. *WHO Report on the Global Tobacco Epidemic: Warning about the Dangers of Tobacco.* Geneva: World Health Organization, 2011.

33. Zhu, X. "STMA: The Increase of Tobacco Tax Did Not Influence the Retail Price Temporarily." *Yangtse Evening Post,* June 22, 2009, http://news.xinhuanet.com /fortune/2009-06/22/content_11578179.htm.

34. Li, C. "The Political Mapping of China's Tobacco Industry and Anti-smoking Campaign." *John L. Thornton China Center Monograph Series* no. 5 (2012), http:// www.brookings.edu/~/media/Research/Files/Papers/2012/10/25%20china%20 tobacco%20li/25%20china%20tobacco%20li.pdf.

35. Gonghuan, Y. "China Wrestles with Tobacco Control." *Bulletin of World Health Organization* no. 88 (2010): 252.

36. Lv, J., M. Su, Z. Hong, T. Zhang, X. Huang, B. Wang, and L. Li. "Implementation of the WHO Framework Convention on Tobacco Control in Mainland China." *Tobacco Control* April 14, 2011, doi:10.1136/tc.2010.040352.

37. Yang, G.-H., Q. Li, C.-X. Wang, J. Hsia, Y. Yang, L. Xiao, J. Yang, L. H. Zhao, J. Zhang, and L. Xie. "Findings from 2010 Global Adult Tobacco Survey: Implementation of MPOWER Policy in China." *Biomedical and Environmental Sciences* 23, no. 6 (2010): 422–9.

38. Li, "The Political Mapping of China's Tobacco Industry."

39. "China Announces New Limits on Smoking in Film and Television." *Telegraph*, February 15, 2011, http://www.telegraph.co.uk/news/worldnews/asia/china /8324848/China-announces-new-limits-on-smoking-in-film-and-television.html.

40. National People's Congress. "Woguo Guomin Jingji He Shehui Fazhan Shi-erwu Guihua Gangyao" [China's 12th Five-Year Plan for National Economic and Social Development]. *People's Daily*, March 17, 2011, http://news.sina.com.cn/c/2011 -03-17/055622129864.shtml.

41. Cheng, L., and Q. Zhong. "China Calls for Tobacco Control Legislation." *People Daily*, March 12, 2014, http://news.xinhuanet.com/english/special/2014-03/12/c _133181392.htm

42. "Harbin to Ban Smoking in Restaurants." *China Daily*, February 22, 2012, http://www.chinadaily.com.cn/china/2012-02/22/content_14671029.htm.

43. Junling, G., C. Simon, S. Shaojing, F. Hua, and Z. Pinpin. "The Growth in Newspaper Coverage of Tobacco Control in China, 2000–2010." *BMC Public Health* 12, no. 1 (2012): 160.

44. "China Announces New Limits on Smoking in Film and Television."

45. Ibid.

46. "China Party School Proposes Stronger Tobacco Control Laws." *Bloomberg News*, December 11, 2013, http://www.bloomberg.com/news/2013-12-11/china-party -school-proposes-stronger-tobacco-control-laws.html.

47. Ibid.

48. "74tian Duohui Liangyi Yuan Yancao Qiye Xiang Shanghai Shiboju Juankuan Beitui" [Recapturing 200 Million RMB in 74 Days: The Endowment to Shanghai Expo Committee from the Tobacco Company Is Returned]. *Health Times*, July 28, 2009, http://health.sohu.com/20090728/n265541593.shtml.

49. Yang et al., "Findings from 2010 Global Adult Tobacco Survey."

50. Jin, "FCTC and China's Politics of Tobacco Control."

51. Song, X. "Zhongguo Kongyan Xiehui Shou Zhiyi" [China Tobacco Control Association Questioned]. *China Gongyi Shibao*, August 23, 2011.

52. World Health Organization. *Global Adult Tobacco Survey (GATS) Fact Sheet China*. Geneva: World Health Organization, 2010.

53. Yang, G. *China Wrestles with Tobacco Control: An Interview with Dr. Yang Gonghuan*. Geneva: World Health Organization, 2010.

54. Ibid.

55. "China Announces New Limits on Smoking in Film and Television."

56. Hu, T. W., Z. Mao, M. Ong, E. Tong, M. Tao, H. Jiang, K. Hammond, K. R. Smith, J. de Beyer, and A. Yurekli. "China at the Crossroads: The Economics of Tobacco and Health." *Tobacco Control* 15, suppl. 1 (2006): 137–41.

57. Jin, "FCTC and China's Politics of Tobacco Control."

58. Li, C. "The Political Mapping of China's Tobacco Industry and Anti-smoking Campaign." *John L. Thornton China Center Monograph Series* no. 5 (2012): 82, http:// www.brookings.edu/~/media/Research/Files/Papers/2012/10/25%20china%20 tobacco%20li/25%20china%20tobacco%20li.pdf.

59. Quan, K. "Jiedu Guowuyuan Dabuzhi Gaige Yu Yancao Gaizhi [Analysis on

the Super Ministerial Reform and Tobacco Industry Reform Formulated by the State Council]." *Tobacco China,* March 13, 2008, http://www.tobaccochina.com/news /analysis/wu/20083/2008312144420_292800.shtml.

60. Yang, L., H. Y. Sung, Z. Mao, T. W. Hu, and K. Rao. "Economic Costs Attributable to Smoking in China: Update and an 8-Year Comparison, 2000–2008." *Tobacco Control* 20, no. 4 (2011): 266–72.

61. Jin, "FCTC and China's Politics of Tobacco Control."

62. Ma, S., interview by author, Los Angeles, CA, February 10, 2014.

Chapter 9 · Conclusion

1. Hoffman, S. J., and J.-A. Røttingen. "A Framework Convention on Obesity Control?" *The Lancet* 378, no. 9809 (2011): 2068.

2. Keck, M. E., and K. Sikkink. *Activists beyond Borders: Advocacy Networks in International Politics.* Ithaca, NY: Cambridge University Press, 1998.

3. Yach, D. "The Origins, Development, Effects, and Future of the WHO Framework Convention on Tobacco Control: A Personal Perspective." *The Lancet* 383, no. 9930 (2014): 1771–9.

4. Taylor, A. L., T. Alfven, D. Hougendobler, S. Tanaka, and K. Buse. "Leveraging Non-binding Instruments for Global Health Governance: Reflections from the Global Aids Reporting Mechanism for WHO Reform." *Public Health* 128, no. 2 (2014): 151–60.

5. Ibid.

6. Ibid.

Page numbers in italics indicate figures.